SpringerWienNewYork

Manfred Wick
Wulf Pinggera
Paul Lehmann

Clinical Aspects and Laboratory – Iron Metabolism, Anemias

Concepts in the anemias of malignancies and renal and rheumatoid diseases

Sixth, revised and updated edition

With contributions by
Volker Ehrhardt

SpringerWienNewYork

Dr. Manfred Wick
Institute of Clinical Chemistry, Klinikum Grosshadern,
University of Munich, Germany

Univ.-Prof. Dr. Wulf Pinggera
Maria Taferl, Austria

Dr. Paul Lehmann
Mainz, Germany

With contributions by
Dr. Volker Ehrhardt
Roche Diagnostics GmbH, Mannheim, Germany

Typesetting: Thomson Press (India) Ltd., Chennai
Printing: Holzhausen Druck GmbH, 1140 Wien, Austria

Printed on acid-free and chlorine free bleached paper
SPIN 12791699

Library of Congress Control Number: 2010942019

With 57 Figures

ISBN 978-3-211-00695-5 5th edn. SpringerWienNewYork
ISBN 978-3-7091-0086-8 SpingerWienNewYork

Foreword

Anemias are a worldwide problem. Severe anemia affects mainly older women and men. The WHO defines anemia as a hemoglobin concentration of less than 12 g/dL in women and less than 13 g/dL in men (World Health Organization. Nutritional Anemias. Technical Reports Series 1992; 503). According to these criteria, 10–20% of women and 6–30% of men above the age of 65 years are anemic. In this book, we place a new emphasis on the diagnosis and treatment of anemias of chronic disease (ACD) and renal anemias. Nevertheless, iron deficiency remains globally the most important cause of anemia.

There have been so many advances in the diagnosis and, in particular, the therapy of the anemias in recent years that it appeared necessary to extend the spectrum of therapies and diagnostic methods described. Apart from renal and inflammatory anemias, new insights regarding the role of transferrin receptor, the physiology of erythropoietin production, and the genetic defect as well as the pathogenesis of hemochromatosis demanded a major update of the book.

The authors are grateful to Annett Fahle and Ralf Röddiger of Roche Diagnostics GmbH for their committed cooperation and their support in the publication of this book.

November 2010

M. Wick
W. Pinggera
P. Lehmann

Table of Contents

Introduction 1

Iron Metabolism 3
  Absorption of Iron 3
  Iron Transport in the Circulation 5
    Transferrin, Iron-Binding Capacity and Transferrin Saturation 5
  Iron Storage – Ferritins, Isoferritins. 8
  Distribution of Iron in the Body 11
  Iron Requirement and Iron Balance 12
    Transferrin Receptor. 12
    Soluble Transferrin Receptor. 14
  Hepcidin 15

Erythropoiesis. 17
  Physiological Cell Maturation 17
  Hemoglobin Synthesis 18
    Erythropoietin. 19
  Erythrocyte Degradation 22
    Phagocytosis of Old Erythrocytes 22
  Hemoglobin Degradation 22

Disturbances of Iron Metabolism/Disturbances
of Erythropoiesis and Hemolysis. 24
  Disturbances of Iron Balance. 24
  Iron Deficiency 25
  Disturbances of Iron Distribution 27
    Anemias of Malignancies and Anemias of Chronic Diseases. 28
  Differentiation between Shortage of Depot Iron
  and Functional Iron Deficiency. 31

Fundamentals

Fundamentals

Disturbances of Iron Utilization 32
    Renal Anemias 32
    Pathophysiology of Erythropoietin Synthesis. 34
Iron Overload. 36
    Primary Hemochromatosis 38
    Other Hereditary States of Iron Overload 39
Other Disturbances of Erythropoiesis. 40
    Disturbances of Stem Cell Proliferation. 40
    Vitamin B_{12} and Folic Acid Deficiency 41
    Hemoglobinopathies 43
    Disturbances of Porphyrin Synthesis. 45
Pathologically Increased Hemolysis 46
    Haptoglobin 47
    Features of Severe Hemolysis. 47
    Causes of Hemolysis (Corpuscular/Extracorpuscular). 48

Diagnosis of Disturbances of Iron Metabolism 50
    Iron Balance 50
    Case History and Clinical Findings 52
    Ferritin, Transferrin, Transferrin Saturation, Soluble Transferrin
    Receptor. 52
    Laboratory Diagnostics of Suspected Disturbances of Iron
    Metabolism. 61
    Most Frequent Disturbances of Iron Metabolism and Erythropoiesis 66
    Hypochromic, Microcytic Anemias. 66

Clinical Aspects

Iron Deficiency – Diagnosis and Therapy 68
    Laboratory Diagnostics in Cases of Suspected Iron Deficiency. 68
    Clinical Pictures of Iron Deficiency 71
    Oral Administration of Iron 74
    Parenteral Administration of Iron 76
    Side-Effects and Hazards of Iron Parenteral Therapy. 78

Disturbances of Iron Distribution and Hypochromic Anemias 80
    Iron and Cellular Immunity 82
    Activation of the Immunological and Inflammatory Systems 85
    Therapy with Erythropoietin and i.v. Iron Administration. 88

Anemias of Infection and Malignancy *91*
Biological Activity of Tumor Necrosis Factor. 92
Hemoglobin in Therapies with Cytostatic Drugs 93
Erythropoietin and Iron Replacement in Tumor Anemias 95
Anemias of Chronic Inflammatory Processes *101*
Anemias of Rheumatoid Arthritis. 102
Erythropoietin and Iron Therapy of Rheumatoid Arthritis. 104

Disturbances of Iron Utilization **106**
Uremic Anemia 106
Therapy of Uremic Anemia 108

Iron Overload **113**
Primary Hematochromatosis 114
Secondary Hematochromatosis 116

Non-Iron-Induced Disturbances of Erythropoiesis **117**

Macrocytic, Hyperchromic Anemia *118*
Folic Acid 120
Vitamin B$_{12}$ 123
Normochromic, Normocytic Anemia. *126*
Extracorpuscular Hemolytic Anemia 128
Corpuscular Anemias 129
Erythropoietin Therapy of Other Diseases. 130

Methods of Determination **132**

Serum/Plasma Parameters *132*
Iron. 133
Iron Saturation (Total Iron-Binding Capacity and Latent
Iron-Binding Capacity). 135
Iron-Binding Proteins. 135
Ferritin 137
Transferrin 140
Transferrin Saturation 141
Soluble Transferrin Receptor. 142
Haptoglobin 142

Clinical Aspects

Laboratory

Ceruloplasmin 144
Vitamin B$_{12}$ 145
Holotranscobalamin 146
Folic Acid 147
Homocysteine. 149
Erythropoietin. 150
Blood Count *151*
Automated Cell Counting 153
Flow Cytometry 153
Impedance-Based Cell Counters 156
Hemoglobin. 158
Hematocrit 159
Red Blood Cell Count 161
Red Blood Cell Indices. 162
Reticulocyte Count 165
Hemoglobin Content of Erythrocytes. 170
Erythrocyte Ferritin. 170
Zinc Protoporphyrin 171
Tests for the Diagnosis of Chronic Inflammation *171*
Erythrocyte Sedimentation Rate 172
C-Reactive Protein 172
Interleukin-6 173
Interleukin-8 174
Tumor Necrosis Factor-α 175

References 176
Further Reading 188
Subject Index 190

Laboratory

Introduction

Disturbances of iron metabolism, particularly iron deficiency and iron redistribution are among the most commonly overlooked or misinterpreted diseases. This is due to the fact that the determination of transport iron in serum or plasma, which used to be the conventional diagnostic test, does not allow a representative estimate of the body's total iron reserves. In the past, a proper estimate was possible only by the costly and invasive determination of storage iron in the bone marrow. However, sensitive, well-standardized immunochemical methods for the precise determination of the iron storage protein ferritin in plasma are now available. Since the secretion of this protein correctly reflects the iron stores in the majority of cases, these methods permit fast and reliable diagnoses, particularly of iron deficiency status. In view of the high incidence of iron deficiency and its usual simple treatment, this fact should be common knowledge in the medical world.

Even non-iron-related causes of anemia can now be identified rapidly by highly sensitive, well-standardized methods. We hope that this book will contribute to a better understanding of the main pathophysiologic relationships and diagnostic principles (Fig. 1) of iron metabo-

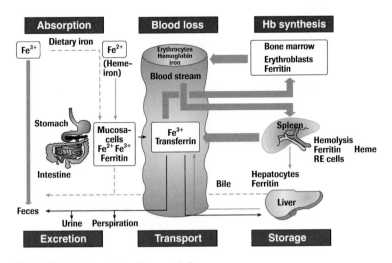

Fig. 1: Physiological principles of iron metabolism

lism and anemias. However, the diagnosis of bone marrow diseases in the strict sense of the word, particularly if granulopoiesis or thrombopoiesis is involved, should remain the responsibility of hematologically experienced experts.

Iron Metabolism

Absorption of Iron

Iron, as a constituent of hemoglobin and cytochromes, is one of the most important biocatalysts in the human body. The absorption of iron by the human body is limited by the physico-chemical and physiologic properties of iron ions, and is possible only through protein binding of the Fe^{2+} ion (Fig. 2).

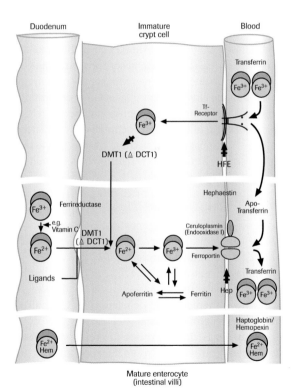

Fig. 2: Intestinal iron absorption
DMT1: Divalent Metal Transporter; DCT1: Divalent Cation Transporter;
Tf: Transferrin; HFE: Hemo-Iron; sTfR: soluble Transferrin Receptor; Hep: Hepcidin

Iron is absorbed as Fe^{2+} in the duodenum and in the upper jejunum. Since iron in food occurs predominantly in the trivalent form it must (apart from the heme-bound Fe^{2+} component) first be reduced e.g. by ascorbic acid (vitamin C). This explains why only about 10% of the iron in food, corresponding to about 1 mg per day, is generally absorbed. This daily iron intake represents only about 0.25‰ of the body's average total iron pool, which is approximately 4 g; this means that it takes some time to build up adequate reserves of iron. The actual iron uptake fluctuates considerably, depending on the absorption-inhibiting and absorption-promoting influences in the upper part of the small intestine. The following factors inhibit absorption in clinically healthy individuals: reduced production of gastric acid, a low level of divalent iron as a result of an unbalanced diet (e.g., in vegetarians), a low level of reducing substances (e.g., ascorbic acid) in the food, or complex formation due to high consumption of coffee or tea. Conversely, absorption is promoted by a combination of a meat-rich diet with a plentiful supply of heme-bound iron and an acidic, reducing environment due to a high consumption of fruit and vegetables. Dietary iron is mostly present either as Fe^{3+} or as heme. Whereas the absorption of heme is less completely characterized by the mechanism of Fe^{3+} absorption has become clearer. It is assumed that it proceeds in two stages. At first, Fe^{3+} is reduced by ferric reductase (duodenal cytochrome b) to Fe^{2+} which is then transported across the cell membrane by a ferrous iron transporter (divalent metal transporter 1, DMT1 or DCT1). In the cells, Fe^{2+} is stored bound to ferritin. Before export into the blood plasma by ferroportin, Fe^{2+} is oxidized to Fe^{3+} by an endooxidase (ceruloplasmin in macrophages, hephaestin in enterocytes). In the plasma, Fe^{3+} is bound to transferrin [62].

The transport protein for iron, DTC1, is mainly localized in the duodenum within the enterocytic membrane and increases in concentration during alimentary iron deficiency. DTC1 is also expressed in the kidneys, liver, brain, and heart [62].

Within certain limits, the absorption of iron can be adjusted to meet the organism's iron requirement. Iron deficiency, anemia, and hypoxia lead via increased transferrin and DCT1 synthesis to an increase in the absorption and transport capacity.

Two models were postulated for the regulation of iron absorption. In the so-called "crypt programming" model, immature crypt cells serve as iron sensors by uptake of Fe^{3+} bound to transferrin via the basolateral membrane with the aid of the transferrin receptor. Essential for the normal function of the transferrin receptor is a protein encoded by the HFE gene. The amount of iron taken up by the immature enterocytes regulates the expression of the iron transporters described above. In case of iron deficiency, more transporters are exprimed; in case of iron overload, the expression of iron transporters is decreased. Consequently, after translocation of the matured enterocytes to the villi, iron absorption depends on the number of iron transporters exprimed in the immature cells.

In the second model, the "iron hormone" hepcidin plays a central role in the regulation of iron recycling and iron balance. Hepcidin is a peptide sythesized by the liver. It inhibits iron uptake in the duodenum and the release of iron from intracellular storage pools. It is assumed that the inhibition of hepcidin is caused by binding to and inducing the degradation of ferroportin, the sole iron exporter in iron-transporting cells. The expression of hepcidin is regulated in response to anemia and hypoxia, and iron load. When oxygen delivery is inadequate, the hepcidin levels decrease and more iron is absorbed in the duodenum, and made available from intracellular iron stores. The opposite occurs with iron load. For the normal regulation of hepcidin levels, the intact HFE gene is required [10].

Iron Transport in the Circulation

Iron is normally transported via the specific binding of Fe^{3+} by transferrin in blood plasma [42]. The Fe^{3+}-transferrin complex in turn is bound by transferrin receptors to cells of the target organs which allow specific iron uptake according to the individual needs of the various cells. Pronounced non-specific binding to other transport proteins, such as albumin, occurs in conditions of iron overload with high levels of transferrin saturation.

When there is an excess supply of heme-bound iron, part of the Fe^{2+}-heme complex may escape oxidation in the cells of the mucosa and be transported to the liver after being bound by haptoglobin or hemopexin.

Transferrin, Iron-Binding Capacity, and Transferrin Saturation

Transferrin (Fig. 3) is the most important and specific iron transport protein in the circulation. It is synthesized in the liver, and has a half-life

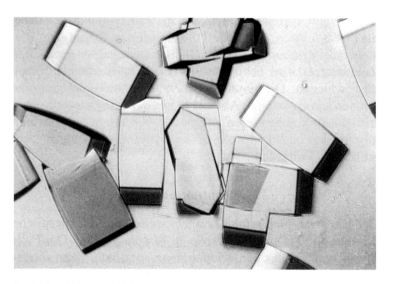

Fig. 3: Transferrin crystals [64]

of 8–12 days in the blood. Transferrin is a glycoprotein with a molecular weight of 79.6 kD, and β_1 electrophoretic mobility. Its synthesis in the liver may be increased as a corrective measure, depending on iron requirements and iron reserves. At present little is known about the details of the regulatory mechanisms involved. Transferrin is detectable not only in blood plasma, but also in many interstitial fluids, and a locally synthesized variant with a low neuraminic acid content (β_2- or τ-transferrin) is found in the cerebrospinal fluid. The functional and immunologic properties of the many isoforms are substantially the same, the only important difference being the isoelectric point [42]. These forms are therefore of no practical interest with regard either to analytical technique or to the assessment of the iron metabolism (except CDT: diagnosis of alcoholism and β_2-transferrin: CSF diagnostics). Each transferrin molecule can bind a maximum of 2 Fe^{3+} ions, corresponding to about 1.41 µg of iron per mg of transferrin.

By measurements of iron and transferrin concentrations, the total specific iron-binding capacity in plasma can be determined. Owing to its practicability, its low susceptibility to interference, and its high specificity, this method should be used to determine the iron transport by

Fundamentals

transferrin. It has made the determination of the iron saturation = total iron-binding capacity (TIBC) and of the latent iron-binding capacity (LIBC) largely redundant.

Under physiologic conditions, transferrin is present in concentrations which exceed the iron-binding capacity normally necessary. The fraction of transferrin-binding sites that are not occupied by iron is known as the latent iron-binding capacity (LIBC). It is calculated from the difference between the total iron-binding capacity and the serum iron concentration.

This procedure has been replaced by the determination of the percentage saturation of transferrin (TfS), which does not include non-specific binding of iron by other proteins, so that only the physiologically active iron binding is measured. Fluctuations of the transferrin concentration that are not due to the regulatory variations of the iron metabolism can also be eliminated from the assessment in this manner.

Approximately one third of the total iron-binding capacity is normally saturated with iron. Whereas the transferrin concentration remains constant in the range from 2.0 to 4.0 g/L, without any appreciable short-term fluctuations, the transferrin saturation changes quickly with the iron concentration depending on the time of day, the current iron requirement, and the intake of dietary iron. The total quantity of transferrin-bound iron in the blood plasma of a healthy adult is only about 4 mg, i.e. only 1‰ of the body's total iron pool of about 4 g.

It is clear from the very low plasma iron concentration and its short-term fluctuations that neither the plasma iron concentration nor the transferrin saturation can provide a true picture of the body's total iron reserves. Assessment of the body's iron reserves is only possible by determination of the storage protein ferritin.

The plasma iron concentration and the transferrin saturation only become relevant in the second stage of diagnosis for differentiation of conditions with high plasma ferritin concentrations (see "Disturbances of Iron Distribution and Iron Overload"). The determination of the transferrin saturation is preferable to the determination of iron alone, since this eliminates the effects of different blood sampling techniques, different states of hydration of the patient, and different transferrin concentrations. Additionally, the determination of the soluble transferrin receptor (sTfR) has gained importance.

Iron Storage – Ferritins, Isoferritins

Because of the very limited iron absorption capacity, the average iron requirement can be met only by extremely economical recycling of active iron. Iron is stored in the form of ferritin or its semi-crystalline condensation product hemosiderin in the liver, spleen, and bone marrow. In principle, every cell has the ability to store an excess of iron through ferritin synthesis. The fundamental mechanisms are identical for all types of cells (Fig. 4).

Iron directly induces the synthesis of apoferritin, the iron-free protein shell of ferritin, on the cytoplasmic ribosomes. In the majority of metabolic situations, a representative fraction of the ferritin synthesized is released into the blood plasma. The ferritin concentration correctly reflects the amount of storage iron available (exception: disturbances of iron distribution). This has been verified experimentally by comparison with iron determinations in bone-marrow aspirates and by monitoring serum ferritin after serial blood donations. In clinical diagnosis, ferritin should be determined as the parameter of first choice for the assessment of iron reserves, e.g. in the identification of the cause of an anemia.

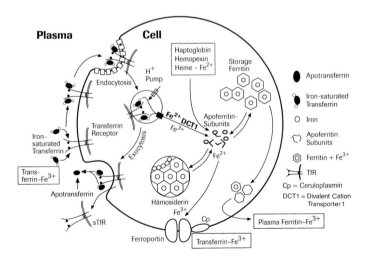

Fig. 4: Scheme of cellular iron storage and ferritin synthesis

The relationship between iron reserves and serum ferritin is valid for all stages of iron deficiency, the normal state, and almost all forms of iron overload. The rule of thumb is:

> **1 ng/mL (µg/L) of serum ferritin corresponds to approximately 10 mg of stored iron.**

This can be used not only to estimate the amount of iron required to replenish stores during iron deficiency but also to estimate iron excess in the case of iron overload as well as for the monitoring of the course of these disorders.

In addition to the general mechanisms of cellular iron storage and uptake, the liver and the spleen also have specialized metabolic pathways. Hepatocytes, for example, can convert haptoglobin-bound or hemopexin-bound hemoglobin-Fe^{2+} or heme-Fe^{2+} from intravascular hemolysis or from increased heme absorption into ferritin-Fe^{3+} storage iron. On the other hand, the regular lysis of senescent erythrocytes and the associated conversion of Fe^{2+}-hemoglobin into Fe^{3+}-ferritin storage iron take place mainly in the reticuloendothelial cells of the spleen. The decisive role in the intracellular oxidation of Fe^{2+} into Fe^{3+} is played by ceruloplasmin.

Ferritin has a molecular weight of at least 440 kD (depending on the iron content), and consists of a protein shell (apoferritin) of 24 subunits and an iron core containing an average of about 2500 Fe^{3+} ions (in liver and spleen ferritin; Fig. 5). Ferritin tends to form stable oligomers (approx. 10–15%), and when present in excess in the cells of the storage organs it tends to condense, with formation of semi-crystalline hemosiderin in the lysosomes.

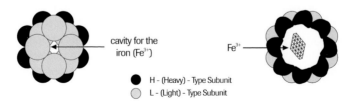

cavity for the iron (Fe^{3+}) Fe^{3+}

● H - (Heavy) - Type Subunit
○ L - (Light) - Type Subunit

Fig. 5: Structure of the ferritin molecule

Seperation behaviour in
isoelectric focusing

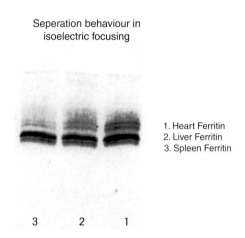

1. Heart Ferritin
2. Liver Ferritin
3. Spleen Ferritin

3   2   1

Fig. 6: Isoelectric focusing of acidic (top) and basic isoferritins (bottom)

At least 20 isoferritins can be distinguished using isoelectric focusing [7] (Fig. 6). The microheterogeneity is due to differences in the contents of acidic H subunits and slightly basic L subunits.

The basic isoferritins are responsible for long-term iron storage, and are found mainly in the liver, spleen, and bone marrow. Plasma ferritin is basic and correlates with the body's total iron stores (exception: disturbances of iron distribution). It can be measured by commercially available immunoassay methods, which are standardized against liver and/or spleen ferritin preparations. Their determination provides a reliable picture of the iron stores. The 3rd International Standard for Recombinant L-Ferritin has been available since 1997 [141].

Acidic isoferritins are found mainly in myocardium, placenta, and tumor tissue, and in smaller quantities also in the depot organs (Table 1). They have lower iron contents, and presumably function as intermediaries for the transfer of iron in synthetic processes [76]. Unlike the basic isoferritins, they exhibit practically no response to the commercially available immunoassay methods. The use of suitable highly specific antisera would be necessary for their selective determination.

Table 1: Clinically important characteristics of the iron storage protein ferritin

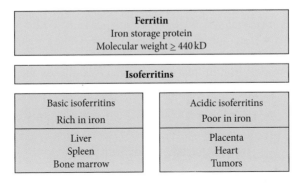

Ferritin
Iron storage protein
Molecular weight $\geq 440\,kD$

Isoferritins

Basic isoferritins	Acidic isoferritins
Rich in iron	Poor in iron
Liver	Placenta
Spleen	Heart
Bone marrow	Tumors

Distribution of Iron in the Body

It can be seen from Fig. 7 that most (about 2500 mg) of the total iron pool is contained in the hemoglobin of the erythrocytes. A further

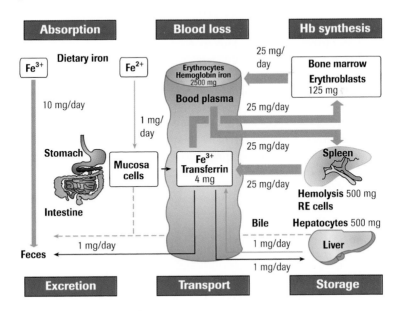

Fig. 7: Balance of iron metabolism

400 mg is contained in myoglobin and various enzymes. If the supply of iron is adequate (men and postmenopausal women), considerable quantities are also stored as basic ferritin (approx. 800–1200 mg) in the depot organs liver, spleen, and bone marrow. Only a small fraction (approx. 4 mg) of the body's total iron pool is in the form of transferrin-bound transport iron in the blood plasma. It is thus once again clear that the measurement of iron in plasma does not provide a true picture of the available storage iron.

Iron Requirement and Iron Balance

The internal turnover of iron resulting from the degradation of senescent erythrocytes, at about 20–25 mg per day, is much higher than the daily intake and excretion of iron. The individual requirement to newly synthesize hemoglobin, myoglobin, and enzymes can therefore be met only by extremely economical recycling of available iron reserves.

Unlike its absorption, the excretion of iron is not actively regulated. Healthy adult men and postmenopausal women lose approximately 1 mg per day under normal conditions via intestine, urine, and perspiration. Menstruating women lose 30–60 mL of blood, containing about 15–30 mg of iron, every month.

The iron requirement is up to 5 mg per day for adolescents, menstruating women, and blood donors, as well as in cases of extreme physical stress due to anabolic processes or iron losses. Pregnant women require additional quantities of iron up to 7 mg per day.

An increased iron requirement cannot always be met by increased absorption, even with an adequate supply of dietary iron. The result is a progressive depletion of the iron stores, which can lead to manifest iron deficiency if the supply of iron remains inadequate over a long period.

Transferrin Receptor

The transferrin receptor (TfR) is a transmembrane, disulfide-linked dimer of two identical subunits that binds and internalizes diferric transferrin, thereby delivering iron to the cell cytosol [142]. TfR is found in

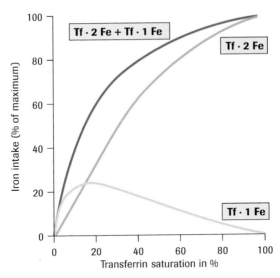

According to HA Huebers et al. (1990)

Fig. 8: Iron uptake by the erythroid progenitor cell in dependency of transferrin saturation [73]

the cytoplasmic membrane of all cells, with the exception of mature erythrocytes. Its molecular weight is about 190 kD. Since the major use of iron is for hemoglobin synthesis, about 80% of total TfR is on erythroid progenitor cells, which have a 10–100-fold higher TfR content than other TfR-containing cells. The membrane-bound receptor on the precursor cells of erythropoiesis is also called the CD71 antigen. The only clearly defined function of the transferrin receptor is to mediate cellular uptake of iron from a plasma glycoprotein, transferrin.

When a transferrin protein loaded with iron ions encounters a transferrin receptor on the cell surface, it binds to it and is consequently transported into the cell in a vesicle. The affinity of the membrane-bound transferrin receptor to the transferrin-Fe^{3+} complex in the weakly alkaline pH of the blood depends on the Fe load of the transferrin. A maximum is reached when transferrin is loaded with $2Fe^{3+}$ ions (Fig. 8). The interior of the endocytotic vesicle acidifies, causing transferrin to release its iron ions into the cytoplasma. The receptor is then transported through the endocytic cycle back to the cell surface, ready for another round of iron uptake (Fig. 9).

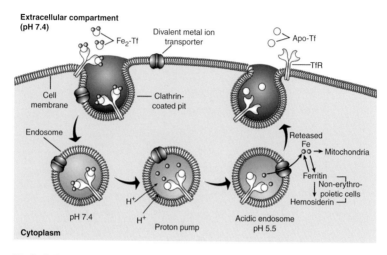

Fig. 9: Cellular iron uptake [5]

The expression of the transferrin receptor is regulated by the intracellular concentration of the iron ions. If the iron requirement of the cell is large, but the iron concentration is small, the expression of TfR increases. Conversely, where there is iron overload, the TfR concentration is low. In most cases, increased erythropoiesis is the main reason for an increased iron requirement. However, it remains to be emphasized that the internal iron demand for Hb-synthesis (25 mg) by far exceeds the average daily absorption of about 1 mg.

The number of transferrin receptors on the erythroid cells increases

- If the iron supply of the functional compartment is inadequate. In this case the erythroid precursor cells produce more TfR.
- In the presence of disease and conditions accompanied by an increase in the mass of erythroid precursor cells, e.g., in the presence of hemolytic anemia. Conditions such as these are identified by an increase in reticulocyte count and the reticulocyte production index.

Soluble Transferrin Receptor

The so-called soluble transferrin receptor (sTfR) is formed by proteolytic cleavage of the transferrin receptor to monomers. It can be quantified

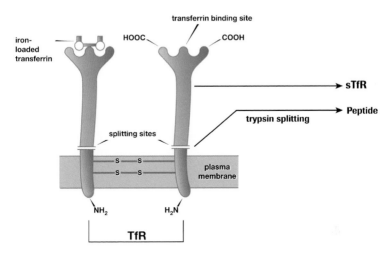

Fig. 10: Schematic view of transferrin receptor and soluble transferrin receptor

by immunochemical methods. As the concentration of the soluble transferrin receptor reflects the total number of cell membrane-bound transferrin receptors [8, 38, 73], and these, in turn, are mainly to be found on erythropoietic cells in the bone marrow, in a healthy person with an adequate iron supply, the soluble transferrin receptor concentration is one of the best indicators of erythropoietic activity [38]. Since the sTfR concentration depends on iron requirement and erythropoietic activity, increased levels of sTfR are found in patients with iron deficient as well as increased erythropoiesis.

Iron deficiency in otherwise healthy persons is relatively easy to diagnose by the determination of ferritin and the soluble transferrin receptor (sTfR). Patients with a chronic disease are more difficult to diagnose, as chronic diseases have a direct effect on the markers of the iron status. In particular, a chronic disease can cause patients with iron deficiency to have normal ferritin values, while the serum iron values can be reduced in patients with sufficient iron reserves. In this group of patients, it has been demonstrated that determination of the soluble transferrin receptor in serum is a valuable alternative to the identification of these patients by Fe determinations in bone-marrow aspirates [117].

Fundamentals

Hepcidin

Human hepcidin is a 25-amino acid peptide first identified in human urine. The main site of synthesis is the liver. The specific role of hepcidin was studied by assessing the effects of its deficiency or excess in transgenic mice. The results of these studies suggest that hepcidin controls extracellular iron by acting as a negative regulator of iron transport in the small intestine and placenta and by inducing iron retention in macrophages. Hepcidin synthesis is increased by iron loading and is decreased by anemia and hypoxia. Since hepcidin is also markedly induced during inflammation, it contributes to the anemia of inflammation. Hepcidin deficiency due to the dysregulation of its synthesis causes most known forms of hemochromatosis.

The applicability of the hepcidin or pro-hepcidin [10] determination in plasma for the diagnostic classification of anemias is not yet clarified. Further studies to validate preanalytic, methodological, and clinical aspects of this parameter are still required [41].

Erythropoiesis

Physiological Cell Maturation

An adult has on average 5 liters of blood and an erythrocyte count of $5 \times 10^6/\mu L$, giving a total erythrocyte count of 2.5×10^{13}. Since the mean life span of an erythrocyte is normally 120 days, about 2×10^{11} new erythrocytes need to be formed daily to maintain this erythrocyte pool. For this to happen, 20–30% of the medullary stem cells must be differentiated to cells of erythropoiesis. Different stages in maturation can be identified on the basis of cell morphology and biochemical capacity. The immature nucleated cells, such as proerythroblasts and erythroblasts (macroblasts), with their high DNA, RNA, and protein synthesizing capacity, ensure that there is adequate proliferation of erythrocyte precursors.

However, this requires the availability of sufficient cobalamin (vitamin B_{12}) and folic acid, which act as carriers of C_1 units in the synthesis of nucleic acids. Vitamin B_{12} (daily requirement about $2 \mu g$) is derived mainly from foods of animal origin. Absorption in the terminal ileum calls for the production of sufficient intrinsic factor by the parietal cells in the fundus/body region of the stomach. By contrast, folic acid (daily requirement $>200 \mu g$) is derived mainly from foods of plant origin and, probably for the most part, via synthesis by intestinal bacteria, and absorbed in the jejunum. Both vitamins are mainly stored in the liver.

Most of the hemoglobin synthesis occurs during the normoblast stage of the erythrocyte precursors. This is morphologically visible by the conversion of so-called basophilic into oxyphilic normoblasts (with red cytoplasm). In parallel, the transferrin receptor is expressed at a high rate which is necessary to channel a sufficient quantity of transferrin-bound iron into the cells.

Cell nucleus and mitochondria are then expelled and the cells leave the bone marrow as reticulocytes. At this stage, the cells' ability to divide and most of their biochemical synthesis capabilities are lost. However, since a considerable amount of Hb-coding mRNA, a high concentration of membrane-bound transferrin receptors, and residual cell organelles persist they are still capable to synhesize Hb for 1–2 days (until mRNA, TfR, and cell organelles are degraded). Within this time about 20% of the mature erythrocyte's Hb is synthesized. Subsequently, the cells circulate in the peripheral blood as highly specialized, mature erythrocytes serving almost exclusively for the transportation of oxygen. This whole process of erythropoiesis takes approximately 5 days.

All forms of anemias that are not primarily hemolytic have their roots in disturbances of cell proliferation or hemoglobin synthesis or in deficiencies at bone-marrow level. The simplest indicator of erythropoiesis is the reticulocyte count.

Hemoglobin Synthesis

In the fetus, hemoglobin (Hb) is made up of 2 α- and 2 γ-polypeptide chains (HbF $(\alpha\gamma)_2$), whereas in adults it predominantly consists of 2 α- and 2 β-chains (HbA$_0$ $(\alpha\beta)_2$), with a small portion of 2 α- and 2 δ-chains (HbA$_2$ $(\alpha\delta)_2$).

Each of these chains carries a heme as prosthetic group, which in turn is capable of binding an oxygen molecule. The total molecular weight of this tetramer is about 64,500 D.

The formation of the normal quaternary structure is dependent on the regular synthesis not only of the peptide chains but also of the heme constituent, and in particular on the adequate adhesion of the heme and protein components by means of iron which also guarantees oxygen binding. An overview of hemoglobin synthesis is given in Fig. 11.

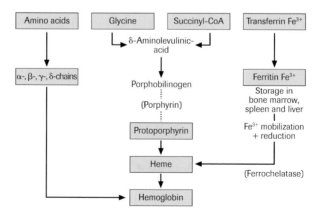

Fig. 11: Hemoglobin synthesis

Erythropoietin

Erythropoietin (EPO) consists of 165 amino acids and has a molecular weight of ~35,000 D (Fig. 12). Approximately 40% of its molecular mass is made up by 4 carbohydrate chains. The hematopoietic growth factor acts synergistically with other growth factors to cause maturation and proliferation from the stage of burst-forming unit erythroid (BFU-E) and CFU-E (colony-forming unit erythroid) to the normoblast stage of erythroid cell development. Thus, EPO acts primarily on apoptosis to decrease the rate of cell death in erythroid progenitor cells in the bone marrow.

During the fetal and neonatal period of life, EPO is primarily produced by the liver. After birth EPO production is shifted to the peri-tubular interstitial cells of the renal cortex. The liver keeps its capability to produce EPO also in the adult, but its contribution is not more than 10%.

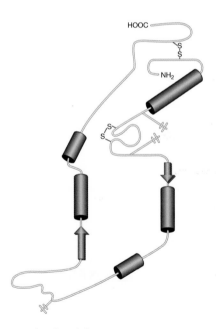

Fig. 12: Molecular structure of erythropoietin

EPO production increases in response to tissue hypoxia, low arterial PO_2, and increased oxygen affinity (HbF) of red blood cells. The hypoxic induction of EPO production is regulated by a negative feedback mechanism at the transcriptional level, which involves binding of HIF-1 (Hypoxia-Inducible Factor-1). HIF-1 acts as an oxygen sensor, which ensures that EPO production is increased when oxygen supply to the tissue is low and the demand for new erythrocytes is high, while EPO production is shut down when red blood cell numbers/and or tissue oxygen supply returns to normal [129]. The characteristics of this control system are depicted in Fig. 13.

Erythropoietin activates target erythroid colony-forming cells by binding and orienting two cell surface erythropoietin receptors. The EPO receptors are primarily expressed on erythroid cells between the CFU-E (Colony-Forming Unit E) and the pronormoblast stages of erythroid cell development. The cell differentiation stages between CFU-E and the pro-erythroblasts have the highest EPO receptor density.

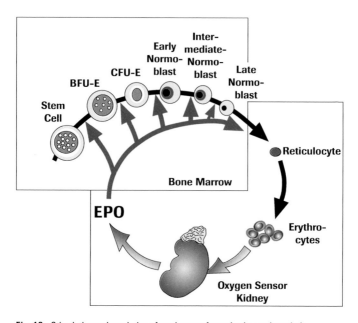

Fig. 13: Stimulation and regulation of erythrocyte formation by erythropoietin

The orientation of the EPO receptors is critical for efficient signaling. Proper binding triggers an intracellular phosphorylation cascade, which activates both the Ras/MAP kinase pathway and the STAT (signal transducer and activator of transcription) pathway. These pathways play a major role in cytokine-induced signaling and are involved in increased cell proliferation in response to EPO [52].

The erythroid progenitor cells are sensitive to EPO and other growth factors for survival, proliferation, and differentiation for only 5 days. The young, just matured erythrocytes require EPO for further 9 days, to prevent their cytolysis in the spleen and the reticuloendothelial system (RES).

In adults, the mean endogeneous EPO level is about $8\,mU/mL$, with a wide range of variation. The strongest stimulus of renal EPO production is an anemic condition. EPO levels typically increase when the level of Hb falls below $12\,g/dL$. By reducing the O_2 transport capacity of Hb, carbon monoxide also leads to a distinct increase of the EPO concentration. Further stimuli of EPO production are an increased affinity of Hb to bind O_2 (HbF), an acceleration of the basal metabolic rate by, e.g. thyroid hormones, benignant and malignant kidney tumors, and a decrease in the O_2 partial pressure in the arterial blood which occurs e.g. with cardiopulmonary illness or deficiency of oxygen in the respiratory air. The stimulation of EPO production by hypoxia is used, e.g. by athletes to increase their erythrocyte count by high altitude training.

An increase of the erythrocyte mass, renal diseases, fasting and resection of the hypophysis lead to a decrease of the EPO production.

Up to now the determination of erythropoietin has been of limited diagnostic value. It can be used, for example, to differentiate between primary causes of erythrocytosis, polycythemia vera and secondary causes such as increased production of erythropoietin, e.g., in lung diseases with hypoxia or certain tumors. In renal anemia, the decreased erythropoietin production can usually be the cause. In every case where a true erythropoietin deficiency does not exist but rather an adequate erythropoietin response, i.e., anemia with normal erythropoietin levels, the determination of erythropoietin is suitable for detecting this inadequate erythropoietin response.

Increased EPO concentrations in serum are measured in patients with cardiac and pulmonary insufficiency, for example, and in patients with erythrocytosis with high oxygen affinity (e.g., HbF). EPO levels typically increase in serum when the Hb level falls below 12 g/dL.

A decrease in EPO concentrations is observed in patients with impaired renal function. Patients with chronic renal insufficiency develop anemia and erythropoiesis is inadequate. Additional extracorporal factors (e.g., hemolysis) can also play a role in the development of anemia.

Erythrocyte Degradation

Phagocytosis of Old Erythrocytes

During the physiologic aging process, the circulating erythrocytes lose more and more of the terminal neuraminic acid residues of their membrane glycoproteins, which leads to increased binding of IgG. The changed membrane surface structure is the signal in particular to the spleen and liver macrophages to start phagocytosis of the aged erythrocytes. About 0.8% of the erythrocyte pool or 2×10^{11} erythrocytes are phagocytozed each day, maintaining equilibrium with the daily new formation rate.

Hemoglobin Degradation

The globin component of the hemoglobin is hydrolyzed by proteases to amino acids which are either available for the synthesis of new proteins or are further degraded. To avoid toxic effects, the released Fe^{2+} is oxidized to Fe^{3+} and incorporated into basic isoferritins for interim storage. In this process, the macrophages of the RES (reticuloendothelial system) in the spleen in particular serve as short-term stores from which ferritin-bound iron can be remobilized and transported via transferrin to the bone marrow for the synthesis of new hemoglobin. At a physiologic hemolysis rate, about 6.5 g per day of hemoglobin is degraded, and the corresponding quantity newly synthesized, giving an iron turnover of about 25 mg/24 h [123, 126]. Given a daily iron absorption of 1 mg, this again shows clearly that the iron requirement can be met only by extensive reutilization.

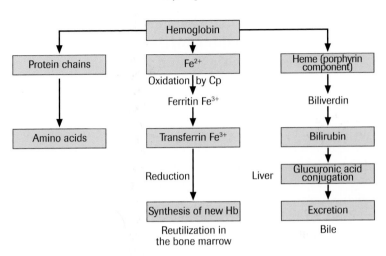

Fig. 14: Hemoglobin degradation
Cp: Ceruloplasmin.

The porphyrin ring of the heme is degraded via biliverdin to bilirubin. Since the unjconjugated bilirubin has poor aqueous solubility it has to be converted into a better water-soluble form to be suited for excretion. For this purpose bilirubin is transported bound to albumin to the liver where it is conjugated with glucuronic acid. The conjugated bilirubin is then excreted with the bile (Fig. 14).

Disturbances of Iron Metabolism/Disturbances of Erythropoiesis and Hemolysis

Disturbances of Iron Balance

An impaired iron balance of the body is frequently recognized by the reverse regulation of synthesis of ferritin, the iron storage protein, on the one hand, and of the transferrin receptor, the indicator of iron demand and erythropoietic activity, on the other. This is particularly true if iron deficiency or iron overload is not complicated by additional diseases such as inflammations, tumors or renal failure (Table 2).

Table 2: Indicators of disturbances of iron balance

	Ferritin	Transferrin saturation	sTfR	Reticulo-cytes	MCV	Hemo-globin
Iron deficiency Latent Manifest	↓ ↓↓	↓ ↓↓	↑ ↑↑	n - ↓ ↓	n - ↓ ↓	n ↓
Iron redistribution (ACD)	n - ↑↑	↓	n - ↑	↓	n - ↓	↓
Renal anemia (without EPO)	n - ↑	↓	n - ↓	↓	n	↓
Iron utilization defects (incl. MDS)	n - ↑	n - ↑	n - ↑	↓	↓ - ↑	↓
Hemolysis	n - ↑	n - ↑	↑	↑	n - ↑	n - ↓
Iron overload (e.g., hereditary hemo-chromatosis)	↑ - ↑↑	↑ - ↑↑	↓	n	n	n

MDS = Myelodysplastic syndrome
ACD = Anemia of chronic disease
n = no change

In true storage iron deficiency a lack of intracellular iron ions leads to downregulation of apoferritin synthesis and consequently also to a decreased release of ferritin into the peripheral blood. To compensate for this, the expression of transferrin receptor is upregulated in order to meet the iron demand of the cell despite depleted iron reserves and low transferrin saturation. This leads to an increased concentration of soluble transferrin receptor in blood. This reverse regulation may be found already in latent iron deficiency, preceding the development of a hypochromic anemia. If these changes are not yet very marked, in doubtful cases the ratio of transferrin receptor and ferritin concentrations may show this state more clearly [117, 138]. The transport iron, determined by measuring the transferrin saturation, additionally contributes to the staging of iron deficiency.

In simple iron overload (for instance hereditary hemochromatosis) the opposite regulation takes place unless the overload is associated with chronic inflammations, malignant disease, ineffective erythropoiesis or hemolysis.

In cases of simple iron overload, the increase of ferritin and downregulation of transferrin receptor production are delayed because the induction of these regulatory processes requires a significant accumulation of intracellular iron. Therefore, particularly in hereditary hemochromatosis increased transferrin saturation is the most sensitive parameter for early detection of iron overload.

The described mechanism of regulation of ferritin and transferrin receptor production is impaired, however, in cases of iron redistribution in chronic inflammations or tumors, in cases of increased erythropoietic activity due to hemolysis or erythropoietin therapy or in bone marrow diseases with increased but ineffective erythropoiesis (for instance myelodysplastic syndrome). This unusual reaction pattern can, however, be used to diagnose an increased iron demand despite sufficient or even increased iron reserves, particularly under erythropoietin therapy.

Iron Deficiency

Even under physiologic conditions, an increased iron requirement and/or increased loss of iron (in puberty, in menstruating or pregnant women, in blood donors or in competitive athletes) can lead to iron deficiency. With an unbalanced diet, the iron balance is often upset by a shortage of absorbable iron.

The first stage is a shortage of depot iron (prelatent iron deficiency), which is reflected in a reduced plasma ferritin concentration. When the iron stores are completely empty, a transport iron deficiency develops, though hemoglobin synthesis is still adequate at this stage (latent iron deficiency). With additional stress or loss of iron, however, this condition may progress into a manifest iron deficiency with hypochromic microcytic anemia. The latter is more often seen with a pathologic chronic loss of blood, especially as a result of ulcers or tumors of the gastrointestinal and urogenital tracts, or with disturbances of iron absorption (e.g., after resections in the upper gastrointestinal tract or chronic inflammatory diseases of the small intestine).

All forms of iron deficiency can be identified by the following pattern of laboratory findings: reduced ferritin concentration with a compensating increase in the transferrin concentration and low transferrin saturation (see "*Diagnostic Strategies*"). The reduced ferritin concentration is the only reliable indicator of iron-deficient conditions. It enables the latter to be distinguished from other causes of hypochromic anemia, such as chronic inflammations and tumors (Table 2).

Iron deficiency, of whatever cause, also leads to increased transferrin receptor expression and accordingly to an increased concentration of the soluble transferrin receptor in the plasma. In these cases, there is no longer any correlation between transferrin receptor and erythropoietic activity. All forms of depot iron deficiency can be detected with an adequate degree of certainty by a decreased ferritin concentration. But since ferritin is an acute phase protein, iron deficiency due to inflammations or tumors may be masked. On the other hand, in cases with sufficient iron reserves and so-called functional iron deficiency, i.e. disturbances of iron utilization, an increased concentration of soluble transferrin receptors may give an early indication of the relative shortage of iron of erythropoiesis or deficient iron mobilization. In these cases of complicated storage or functional iron deficiency, sTfR may show the increased iron demand.

A correct diagnosis of iron deficiency is critical for the successful treatment of anemias. Experience shows that in multimorbid patients iron deficiency can often only be classified as "certain", "absent", or "possible". Patients classified in the latter category primarily have anemias that occur in conjunction with infections, acute chronic inflammation, or malignant tumors. A majority of these patients have an acute phase reaction with increased CRP (C-reactive protein) to above 5 mg/L.

The objective to laboratory testing is to:

- Detect the subclinical iron deficiency and administer early therapy to prevent systemic complications of this disease;
- Identify anemias that are based on uncomplicated iron deficiency (menstruation increased, chronic intestinal bleeding, nutritive iron deficiency), because they respond very quickly to iron therapy;
- Detect inadequate iron supply of erythropoiesis in anemias where disturbance of iron distribution is paramount (anemias in infections and inflammations, and tumor anemia).

Disturbances of Iron Distribution

Malignant neoplasias and chronic inflammations lead to a shortage of transport and active iron, with simultaneous overloading of the iron stores. When tumors are present, the disturbance of the iron distribution is further influenced by the increased iron requirement of the tumor tissue. These conditions, like manifest iron deficiency, are characterized by anemia, low iron levels and low transferrin saturation values. Genuine iron deficiency is distinguished by reduced ferritin and elevated transferrin concentrations.

The elevated ferritin concentration in these cases is not representative of the body's total iron reserves, but indicates the redistribution to the iron-storing tissue. The low transferrin saturation distinguishes disturbances of iron distribution from genuine iron overload conditions.

In the presence of tumors, besides a disturbed iron distribution and increased release of iron-rich basic isoferritins into the blood plasma, a separate release of mainly acidic iron-poor isoferritins is observed. Only a small fraction of the acidic isoferritins is normally detected by commercially available immunoassay methods. Therefore, in most cases the total ferritin concentration is underestimated in the presence of tumors. What is recorded is mainly the redistribution of iron, and to a smaller extent the autochthonous tumor synthesis products.

A non-representative elevation of the plasma ferritin concentration is also found in patients with cell necrosis of the iron-storage organs, e.g. in liver diseases. Transferrin saturation is also elevated in these patients, however.

In most of the iron distribution disturbances, there is a relative shortage in the amount of iron supplied to the erythropoietic cells, together with reduced erythropoietic activity. Correspondingly, transferrin receptor expression is usually normal. However, in the case of rapidly growing tumors, transferrin receptor expression can be elevated as a result of the increased iron requirement of the tumor cells.

A very rare hereditary form of iron redistribution is caused by atransferrinemia. The lack of transferrin-bound iron transport leads to low iron concentrations in plasma and a reduced supply of all iron consuming cells. The transport function is taken over nonspecifically by other proteins such as albumin, leading to an uncontrolled deposition of iron in the cells, which is not regulated according to the demand by transferrin receptor expression.

Anemias of Malignancies and Anemias of Chronic Diseases

As described above, iron redistribution with a relative overloading of iron stores and concomitant relative iron deficiency of erythropoietic cells (as a consequence of reduced transferrin synthesis) can be seen mainly with tumor anemias and chronic inflammations (primarily rheumatic diseases, but also infections). If the disturbance of iron redistribution is predominant, hypochromic anemia is highly probable and can be differentiated from iron deficiency anemia by assaying ferritin and sTfR.

The synthesis of the anti-acute phase protein transferrin is downregulated in the presence of the above-mentioned diseases, which is possibly the result of an evolutionary natural selection process. Suscibility to infections decreases in the presence of reduced transport iron, because bacteria and other pathogens also require iron to replicate. The reduced availability of iron therefore acts as a protective mechanism on the one hand and, on the other, it represents a major pathomechanism of the development of anemias of infection and malignancy.

Apart from downregulation of transferrin production, a second cause of iron redistribution in inflammations was identified [36].

Fundamentals

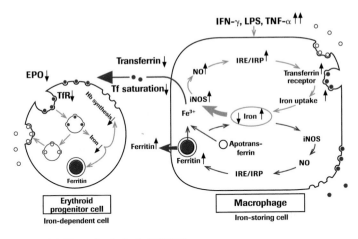

Fig. 15: Model of iron redistribution in ACD [151]

IFN-γ, interferon γ; iNOS, inducible nitric oxide synthase; IRE, iron-responsive element; IRE/IRP high-affinity binding of iron-regulatory protein (IRP) to IREs; LPS, lipopolysaccharide; NO, nitric oxide; TNF-α, tumor necrosis factor α; ↑ and ↓ indicate increase or decrease of cellular responses; respectively. ∪ transferrin receptor; ● iron-carrying transferrin; O apotransferrin; ⊙ ferritin.

Cytokines IFN-γ and TNF-α, mediated by nitric oxide (NO), stimulate iron uptake by macrophages by increased transferrin receptor expression. The increased iron uptake induces ferritin synthesis, which in turn causes enhanced ferritin release into the plasma. The increased iron storage in macrophages of patients with Anemias of Chronic Diseases (ACD) and tumors draws iron from transferrin, which is already reduced. In contrast to true iron overload this kind of iron redistribution is characterized by low transferrin saturation. This mechanism increases the iron deficiency in all iron consuming cells in the body (Fig. 15).

Recently an iron-retentive effect of increased hepcidin levels has been discovered, especially with bacterial, but also parasitic and fungal infections. The retention of iron with the resulting decrease in transferrin saturation leads, together with the already described reduction of the transferrin levels, to a withdrawal of iron not only from the pathogens but also from erythropoiesis [10]. The increased hepcidin production in acute phase reactions is normally self-limiting since the resulting decreased transferrin saturation leads to a downregulation of the expression of the peptide. Hepatic tumors which excessively produce hepcidin seem to be an exception here.

A further cause of ACD results from reduced erythropoiesis due to the inadequate erythropoietin response to anemia and tissue hypoxia [60, 102]. In contrast to renal anemia, this is a possibly cytokine-mediated dysregulation preventing the termination of anemia by increased erythropoietin synthesis. Additionally, erythropoietin effects are reduced. Comparable to absolute erythropoietin deficiency this functional relative erythropoietin deficiency can be substituted with iron and erythropoietin.

In certain cases a hemolytic component also contributes to pathogenesis of anemia, for example due to autoantibodies in the context of a malignant systemic disease or an autoimmune disease.

If hemolysis or a reduced erythropoietin response is the predominant factor in the pathogenesis of the ACD, then the anemia may be normocytic in character rather than microcytic. In the case of marked hemolysis, the reticulocyte count is in the normal to elevated range. If, in contrast, iron redistribution and diminished erythropoietic activity is predominant then a lowered reticulocyte count and microcytic anemia are to be expected.

The pathomechanisms responsible for tumor anemia or anemia of chronic inflammations described above, such as downregulation of transferrin production, iron redistribution into macrophages, and insufficient erythropoietin response fulfill a biologic purpose in the pathogenesis also of tumor anemias. The tumor cells are growth-inhibited by iron depletion which, however, is bought at the expense of an anemia. The iron depletion of erythropoiesis is reflected in the elevated concentration of soluble transferrin receptor, especially in patients with concomitant iron deficiency or after administration of EPO.

Furthermore, in malignant diseases of the hematopoietic system induction of autoantibodies (e.g., cold agglutinins) and splenomegaly may contribute to increased hemolysis, which, as a long-term effect, leads to an iron overload in addition to iron redistribution.

In all malignant diseases and hematologic systemic diseases such as leukemias and lymphomas, an infiltration of the bone marrow by malignant cells associated with a reduction of not only erythropoiesis but also hematopoiesis in general may be important. This is the prognostically most unfavorable form of a tumor anemia with respect to responsiveness to substitution of iron and erythropoietin. This is also true for my-elodysplastic syndromes in which an increased but ineffective erythropoiesis is characterized by a maximal stimulation of erythropoietin production which finally leads to an iron overload state. These bone marrow diseases can be diagnosed adequately only by bone marrow investigation by hematologically experienced experts.

Anemias of gastrointestinal tumors and inflammations (celiac disease, M. Crohn, Colitis ulcerosa, stomach and colon carcinomas) represent exceptional cases of anemias of chronic disease (ACD). In addition to the mechanisms of iron redistribution and reduced erythropoietin response outlined above a deficiency of iron, nutrients, vitamins, and trace elements caused by anorexia, blood loss, diarrhea, and disturbances of iron resorption may play a role here. Since an acute phase reaction associated with non-representative ferritin values is often observed in these cases, the diagnosis can be improved by the additional determination of sTfR and, if necessary, with the assessment of the sTfR/log ferritin ratio [138]. Also in this particular situation, increased sTfR concentrations indicate either an accelerated erythropoiesis with increased iron demand or a shortage of depot iron. The same applies to a lesser extent for diseases of the urogenital tract.

Differentiation between Shortage of Depot Iron and Functional Iron Deficiency

As already outlined, disturbances of iron mobilization and distribution with reduced transferrin saturation and inadequate iron supply (functional iron deficiency) may occur albeit sufficient depot iron. Especially when associated with an acute phase reaction, this situation may be recognized only conditionally by biochemical testing. Reduced transferrin saturation with normal to increased ferritin and normal to decreased sTfR may be indicative here. In this situation the additional determination of cellular indices, especially of the percentage of hypochromic erythrocytes (% HYPO) or the reticulocyte hemoglobin content (Ret-Hb) has gained increased importance [28] for the sensitive detection of an insufficient iron supply of erythropoiesis. The combination of Ret-Hb and sTfR/log ferritin in a diagnostic diagram with CRP concentration-dependent cut-off values may considerably facilitate the differenciation between shortage of depot iron and functional iron deficiency [139].

However, sensitivity and specificity of the cellular indices may be hampered by symptoms of malnutrition (e.g., hypochromia caused by hypoproteinosis, hyperchromia caused by folate or vitamin B_{12} deficiency) or cytostatic therapy (e.g., macrocytosis and hyperchromia caused by treatment with folic acid antagonists).

Disturbances of Iron Utilization

Even with normal serum ferritin concentrations indicative for normal iron reserves and normal iron distribution, disturbances of iron utilization or incorporation can occur. This situation may also lead to microcytic or normocytic anemia, simulating the presence of iron-deficiency anemia.

Ever since erythropoietin has replaced the transfusions previously used to treat renal anemia, dialysis patients represent the largest group. Despite adequate iron reserves, erythropoietin therapy does not always lead to a sufficient iron mobilization from the iron stores. This is demonstrated, e.g. by a reduction in transport iron (low transferritin saturation). Similarly, as in genuine iron deficiency and disturbances of iron distribution, the reduced availability of iron for heme synthesis leads to an increased incorporation of zinc into the porphyrin ring. This can be measured as increased Zn-protoporphyrin in the erythrocytes, and can be used as an additional aid to the diagnosis of iron utilization disturbances with normal or elevated ferritin concentrations. Ferritin and sTfR are suitable means to distinguish between genuine iron deficiency and disturbances of iron distribution or utilization.

Renal Anemias

Particular attention should be paid to iron metabolism in patients with renal anemia. The substitution of erythropoietin, together with the i.v. administration of iron, has replaced transfusions which used to be performed routinely, and has therefore revolutionized therapy.

Transfusions, which previously were performed on a regular basis and the concomitant disturbance of iron utilization due to erythropoietin deficiency almost invariably led to increasing iron overload and its associated consequences. The treatment of disturbances of iron metabolism in dialysis patients is now fundamentally different since the introduction of EPO therapy, however.

The iron reserves are usually adequate, i.e. the plasma ferritin concentration is normal or possibly even increased. Despite normal iron reserves, iron mobilization is typically disturbed. This is indicated by low transferrin saturation, which can lead to relative short supply of iron in erythropoiesis and to so-called functional iron deficiency. Generally this situation cannot be remedied by oral iron replacement therapy as, in most cases, iron absorption is also disturbed.

However, as long as the erythropoietin deficiency typical of renal anemia is not corrected, the erythropoietic activity is reduced to the same extent as the mobilization of iron. Therefore at a low level, iron turnover and erythropoiesis are in a steady state. Transferrin receptor expression is reduced or normal.

Renal anemia can also be complicated, for example, by a hemolytic component as a result of mechanical damage of the red cells during hemodialysis. If this is the case, a normal or even elevated reticulocyte count is to be expected, and not reduced hematopoiesis, as with simple erythropoietin deficiency. In this situation the short supply of iron in erythropoiesis is reflected in the elevated proportion of hypochromic erythrocytes and hypochromic reticulocytes.

If attempts are made to correct the erythropoietin deficiency by substitution, thereby increasing erythropoietic activity, the poor mobilization of the iron reserves is apparent as a functional iron deficiency. The cells of erythropoiesis react by increased expression of the transferrin receptor to improve iron provision. The ferritin concentration is generally a true reflection of the iron reserves (an exception to this is when it is immediately preceded by iron substitution or in the presence of a secondary disorder involving iron distribution disturbances) and can therefore be used to recognize any depot iron deficiency or to avoid iron overload in iron substitution therapy.

Transferrin saturation is currently the best indicator for the amount of mobilizable transport iron and is inversely proportional to the iron requirement. Reduced transferrin saturation in dialysis patients is a sign

Table 3: Assessment of iron metabolism in dialysis patients

Iron reserves	Transport iron
Ferritin	*Transferrin saturation*
Generally adequate or elevated (due to transfusions, Fe replacement, and disturbed Fe mobilization).	Currently best indicator for mobilizable iron.
Iron absorption	**Iron requirement**
(Fe absorption test)	*Soluble transferrin receptor (sTfR)*
Generally abnormal, therefore i.v. Fe administration if required	

of inadequate iron mobilization and therefore of a functional iron deficiency requiring iron substitution (Table 3).

It is possible to use the concentration of the soluble transferrin receptor as a direct indicator of the iron requirement. However, on no account can the transferrin receptor replace the ferritin determination for assessing the iron reserves as it only reflects the current erythropoietic activity and/or its iron requirement, which do not necessarily correlate with the iron reserves [72]. Determination of the zinc protoporphyrin in the erythrocytes has no advantage over the parameters mentioned. Because of the 120-day life span of the erythrocytes, this determination would only reflect the iron metabolism situation at a too late stage.

Pathophysiology of Erythropoietin Synthesis

In progressive renal disease, erythropoietin-producing cells in peritubulary capillaries lose their production capacity leading to a breakdown of the autoregulatory loop which normally guarantees a constant hemoglobin concentration [51]. In patients with renal disease this state, when combined with disturbed iron mobilization, can usually be assumed to be the cause of the anemia. Confirmation by determination of erythropoietin is necessary only in doubtful cases (Table 4).

An insufficient erythropoietin response, probably due to cytokine effects, is probably one of the major causes of tumor anemia and anemia of chronic inflammations. Absolute erythropoietin concentrations are

Table 4: Erythropoietin (EPO), ferritin, and soluble transferrin receptor concentrations in anemias and erythrocytosis

Disease	EPO concentration	Ferritin concentration	sTfR concentration
Anemias			
Iron deficiency	↑	↓	↑
Renal anemia	↓-↓↓	n-↑	n-↓
Anemia of chronic disease	n-↓	n-↑↑	n-↑
Hemolysis	↑	n-↑	↑-↑↑
Bone marrow diseases with ineffective erythropoiesis	↑	↑-↑↑	n-↑
Erythrocytosis			
Reactive hypoxia	↑	variable	↑
Paraneoplastic (e.g. kidney, liver carcinoma)	↑↑	n-↑	↑↑
Polycythemia vera	n-↓	n-↑	↑-↑↑

frequently found to be within the reference range for clinically healthy persons; however, this can be considered to be inadequate in patients with anemia. Inadequate erythropoietin secretion and efficacy and the corresponding iron redistribution can, however, be corrected by erythropoietin and iron therapy, as in renal anemia.

In contrast to these diseases caused by erythropoietin deficiency or insufficient response (Table 4), all other anemias lead to an increased erythropoietin production. This is true for very different causes of anemia, for instance iron deficiency anemia, hemolytic anemias, and many bone marrow diseases with inefficient erythropoiesis. In severe bone marrow damage (for instance aplastic anemia, myelodysplasia) this compensatory mechanism is not effective anymore because the erythroid progenitor cells are missing or fail to mature.

Increased erythropoietin secretion may lead to a secondary erythrocytosis, provided a sufficient iron supply and normal bone marrow function are present. In hypoxia (cardiopulmonary diseases, heavy smokers, staying at high altitude) this is a mechanism of adaptation to oxygen deficiency. In rare cases, however, carcinomas of the kidney or the liver may produce erythropoietin which also leads to erythrocytosis. In contrast to these secondary forms of erythrocytosis, polycythemia vera is an autonomous proliferation of erythroid cells which leads to a compensatory downregulation of erythropoietin production. Determination of erythropoietin can therefore contribute to the differential diagnosis of erythrocytosis in doubtful cases.

Iron Overload

Genuine iron overload situations arise either through a biologically inappropriate increase in the absorption of iron despite adequate iron reserves, or iatrogenically as a result of frequent blood transfusions or inappropriate iron therapy.

The former condition occurs mainly as a result of the disturbance of negative feedback mechanisms, which in hemochromatosis is manifested as a failure of the protective mechanism in the mucosa cell (see "Absorption of Iron").

Conditions characterized by ineffective erythropoiesis, such as thalassemia, porphyrias, and sideroachrestic as well as hemolytic anemias, lead to increased synthesis of erythropoietin, transferrin receptor, and absorption of iron, despite adequate iron reserves (utilization of iron to synthesize hemoglobin is impaired). The iron overload in these cases is aggravated by the necessary transfusions and by the body's inability to actively excrete iron. All the mechanisms mentioned ultimately lead to overloading of the iron stores, and hence redistribution to the parenchymal cells of many organs, such as the liver, heart, pancreas, and gonads. The storage capacity of ferritin or of the lysosomes may thus be exceeded and free iron ions are released into the cytoplasma. The free iron ions can lead to the formation of oxygen radicals which then exert their toxic effects.

The main manifestations in the affected organs are liver cirrhosis and primary liver cell carcinoma, heart failure, diabetes or impotence. Phagocytosis and oxidative burst of granulocytes and monocytes may be impaired as well. Epidemiologic investigations have revealed even latent iron overload to be a risk factor for atherosclerosis and type 2 diabetes due to, among other causes, increased oxidation of low-density lipoproteins (LDL) and the formation of foam cells [54, 143] (Fig. 16).

This calls for an increased surveillance of iron overload in the latent phase already by regular ferritin (warning limit: 400 mg/mL) and sTfR

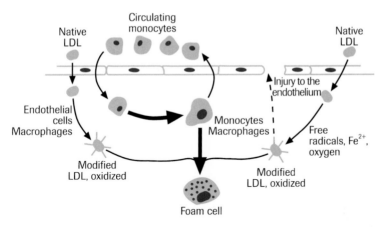

Fig. 16: Effect of iron overload on the oxidation of low-density lipoproteins and the formation of foam cells

determinations. This is true not only for patients with primary hemochromatosis or secondary hemosiderosis and hematologic disease but also in patients with renal anemia or anemia of chronic disease under erythropoietin and iron substitution.

Almost all genuine iron overload conditions are recognizable by elevated plasma ferritin concentrations together with elevated iron levels and increased transferrin saturation values, usually with a compensating decrease in transferrin synthesis. The increased transferrin saturation, as a sign of increased iron turnover and iron transport, distinguishes iron overload from conditions with redistribution of iron and non-representatively raised plasma ferritin concentrations.

Transferrin receptor expression can vary, depending on the reason for the iron overload, in particular whether erythropoiesis is increased or decreased. Correspondingly there is also an elevated transferrin receptor concentration in the plasma in all hemolytic conditions with raised erythropoietic activity.

Contrary to this, all bone marrow disorders with reduced erythropoiesis such as aplastic anemia and also renal failure (without erythropoietin therapy) are characterized by reduced transferrin receptor expression. Erythropoiesis is not directly affected in hemochromatosis. Transferrin receptor expression may be normal or decreased.

Primary Hemochromatosis

Primary hemochromatosis represents the most important form of hereditary iron overload. Until recently its significance has been underestimated but nevertheless a close association between primary hemochromatosis and certain HLA patterns has been known for a long time. Two mutations of the HFE gene were discovered in the majority of white patients with hemochromatosis in the homozygous or compound heterozygous form. The cys-282-tyr mutation is by far the most common mutation and is present in homozygous form in almost 100% of Scandinavian and as many as 69% of Italian hemochromatosis patients. The less common variant is the his-63-asp mutation. Both variations together represent probably the most common of all genetic defects. In the Caucasian population the frequency of the heterozygous defect is 1:15 and that of the homozygous from 1:200 to 1:300. These mutations can routinely be detected by using PCR analysis.

Obviously the mutations give rise to abnormal HFE proteins in the epithelial cells of the mucosa of the small intestine in the region which is relevant for iron absorption. The mutated HFE proteins are not capable to bind to transferrin receptor 2 and the binding of Fe^{3+} to transferrin at high transferrin saturation is compromised (*see "Absorption of Iron"*).

More recent findings indicate that the abnormal HFE proteins also affect the liver. They prevent the upregulation of hepcidin production, which is normally necessary in the case of iron overload. Thereby, the direct inhibiting effect of hepcidin on the transfer of iron from the intestinal cells and macrophages to transferrin is missing [113].

More rare cases of hereditary hemochromatosis have been linked to mutations in the genes encoding hepcidin, hemojuvelin, transferrin receptor 2, and ferroportin. The mechanisms underlying the effects of the genetic variants of hemojuvelin, transferrin receptor 2, and ferroportin are not yet fully understood [113].

Not all patients who have a homozygous gene defect actually develop manifest hemochromatosis. The frequency of hemochromatosis in the Caucasian population is in the order of 1:1000 to 1:2000. This is probably primarily due to the fact that the precondition for clinical manifestation of hemochromatosis is iron overloading of approximately 10–20 g corresponding to serum ferritin values of approximately

1000–2000 ng/mL. Assuming a positive iron balance of approximately 1 mg per day (2 mg absorption and 1 mg excretion) the time required for the accumulation of an excess of iron reserves is approximately 30–60 years. This correlates well with the main age of manifestation of hemochromatosis in men (35–55 years of age). Although the homozygous gene defect is more commonly found in women than men, women are mostly protected from the development of hemochromatosis until the onset of menopause. This is due to the fact that the excess iron absorption is approximately compensated for by iron loss of the same order of magnitude (15–30 mg) in the course of menstrual bleeding. Therefore the process of iron accumulation and iron overloading in women with homozygous hemochromatic genes commences only at the onset of menopause and (compared to the process occurring in men) is delayed by decades into old age. Accordingly only about 10% patients with symptomatic hemochromatosis are women. In an evolutionary context the hemochromatic genes probably represent a natural selection advantage because they protect women against severe iron deficiency until at least the onset of menopause. Only after the achievement of a significantly longer life-expectancy does iron accumulation may prove to be disadvantageous.

Also patients with hetereozygous forms of hemochromatosis store increased amounts of iron. However, in most of these cases a clinical manifestation of iron overload is not seen.

The genetic defects can now be identified in the course of routine diagnostic procedures. Following analysis of ferritin and sTfR concentrations and particularly transferrin saturation PCR detection of the appropriate mutation represents the second level in hematochromatosis diagnostics. However, assaying for ferritin remains the decisive determination for the monitoring of iron reserves.

Other Hereditary States of Iron Overload

The copper transport protein *ceruloplasmin* seems to be important for intracellular oxidation of Fe^{2+} to Fe^{3+} which is necessary for the release of iron ions from the cells and the binding to transferrin. This is indicated by the very rare hereditary aceruloplasminemia where the lack of iron oxidation prevents binding to transferrin and thereby leads to intracellular trapping of iron ions and consequently to the development of an iron overload which resembles hereditary hemochromatosis. However, in contrast to hemochromatosis the central nervous system is also affected. Due to the impaired binding of iron to transferrin, however, iron concentrations and transferrin saturation in plasma are not elevated, whereas ferritin concentrations are high, reflecting the impaired iron distribution and release from the cells.

In the so-called "African dietary iron overload" the increased dietary iron intake from excessive consumption of beer home-brewed in iron drums was long considered the only cause of this iron overload disorder resembling hemochromatosis. However, a non-HLA-linked gene has now additionally been implicated which, as in hemochromatosis, may impair the protective mechanism in the mucosal cells.

Other Disturbances of Erythropoiesis

Disturbances of Stem Cell Proliferation

Even at stem-cell level, physiologic cell maturation can be compromised by numerous noxae and deficiencies, which in this case leads not only to anemia, but also to disturbances of myelopoiesis and thrombocytopoiesis. Examples that can be cited are medullary aplasia induced by autoimmune (e.g., thymoma), infectious (e.g., hepatitis) or toxic (e.g., antineoplastic drugs and benzene) processes or ionizing radiation. Chemical noxae or irradiation can, however, also lead to hyperregenerative bone-marrow insufficiency (myelodysplasia) with iron overload and a possible transition to acute leukemia. Whereas the above-mentioned diseases can be adequately diagnosed only by invasive and costly bone-marrow investigations, the causes of vitamin deficiency-induced disturbances of the proliferation and maturation of bone-marrow cells with macrocytic anemia can be detected more simply by the determination of vitamin B_{12} and folic acid in the serum. However, the differentiation of MDS (myelodysplastic syndrome) and vitamin B_{12}, and folic acid deficiency may be difficult due to similar megaloblastic alterations in bone marrow and macrocytic anemia in all these cases.

Vitamin B₁₂ and Folic Acid Deficiency

Since the very low daily cobalamin requirement of about $2\,\mu g$ can be easily covered with a normal, varied diet, diet-induced vitamin B_{12} deficiency is rare, except in radical vegetarians. The vast majority of deficiency syndromes are therefore caused either by a deficiency of intrinsic factor (chronic atrophic gastritis, gastric resection, antibodies to intrinsic factor) or by disturbances of absorption (fish tapeworm and intestinal diseases). By contrast, folic acid deficiency arises mainly as a result of unbalanced diet and reduced storage in liver damage, especially in connection with alcoholism. Other important causes are malabsorption in intestinal diseases and inhibition of the folic acid synthesis of intestinal bacteria by antibacterial or cytotoxic chemotherapy with folic acid antagonists. The intracellular bioavailability of the active form tetrahydrofolic acid also depends on an adequate supply of vitamin C (reduction) and in particular of vitamin B_{12} (intracellular uptake). Since, for this reason and on account of the transfer of C1 units, folic acid and vitamin B_{12} act synergistically in DNA synthe-

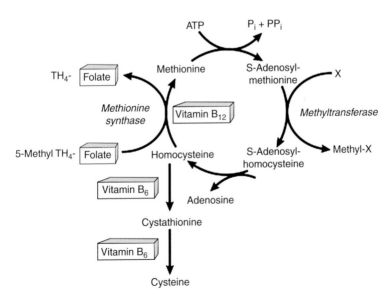

Fig. 17: Metabolism of homocysteine, folate, vitamin B_{12}, vitamin B_6

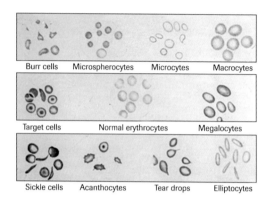

Burr cells   Microspherocytes   Microcytes   Macrocytes

Target cells   Normal erythrocytes   Megalocytes

Sickle cells   Acanthocytes   Tear drops   Elliptocytes

Fig. 18: Normal and pathologic forms of erythrocytes

sis and cell maturation (Fig. 17). Deficiencies similarly lead to macrocytic anemia. On account of the reduced proliferation capacity, especially of the cells of erythropoiesis, the total count of erythrocytes is then significantly reduced. However, since the hemoglobin synthesis capacity is at the same time normal, the individual erythrocytes are not only abnormally large ("macrocytes", Fig. 18) but also have elevated hemoglobin content ("hyperchromic anemia"). In view of the fact that the forms of anemia are the same and that folic acid is active only with an adequate vitamin B_{12} supply, a first diagnosis of macrocytic anemia requires the simultaneous determination of vitamin B_{12} and folic acid and possibly the exclusion of MDS.

If folic acid deficiency is suspected, then the serum folic acid concentration may be in the lower reference range. This can indicate a latent folic acid deficiency which can possibly be proven by determining the folic acid content of erythrocytes or homocysteine [13]. If serum concentrations are normal but the erythrocytes are nevertheless supplied with an insufficient amount of folic acid then an uptake disorder is manifest which is most often caused by a vitamin B_{12} deficiency.

Latent vitamin B_{12} and folic acid deficiency have also received attention. Manifestations of this latent vitamin deficiency prior to the appearance of anemia or funicular spinal disease in vitamin B_{12} deficiency can lead to other metabolic anomalies such as hyperhomocysteinemia, with an elevated risk of neural tube defects, immune deficiencies, and atherosclerosis.

Recently the term "metabolic" vitamin B_{12} or folic acid deficiency has been introduced. It is characterized by the presence of deficiency symptoms (predominantly macrocytic anemia) already at vitamin B_{12} or folic acid concentrations in the lower reference range, possibly due to an increased demand sometimes in the context of MDS or neoplasia. This may be confirmed by further laboratory investigations. Latent or functional folic acid deficiency leads to hyperhomocysteinemia, latent and functional vitamin B_{12} deficiency mainly to an increased concentration and excretion of methylmalonic acid and possibly also of homocysteine. Vitamin B_{12} deficiency can be considered very unlikely, however, if the serum concentration is above 300 ng/L. This is also true for folic acid concentrations within a functionally defined reference range above 4.4 ng/mL.

Hemoglobinopathies

Hemoglobinopathies are a disturbance in the synthesis of the protein components of hemoglobin [32]. A distinction is made between point mutations with exchange of individual amino acids and defects in whole protein chains.

Of the former, sickle-cell anemia is the most important because it is widespread in the black population of Africa and America. The substitution of valine for glutaminic acid at position 6 in the β-chain leads to the formation of so-called sickle-cell hemoglobin (HbS). The HbS molecules tend to aggregate after unloading oxygen. They form long, rod-like structures that force the red cells to assume a sickle shape. Unlike normal red cells, which are usually smooth and deformable, the sickle red cells (Fig. 18) cannot squeeze through small blood vessels. They are visible under the microscope and can therefore be used diagnostically. HbS can also be detected by hemoglobin electrophoresis. Today, this genetic defect is mostly diagnosed using PCR.

Hemoglobinopathies in the broader sense also include the so-called thalassemias. Thalassemia represents a condition in which there is reduced synthesis or complete absence of entire chains from the hemoglobin molecule. Quantitative changes in the synthesis of the α- and β-chains are of particular clinical significance, as these make up HbA, the main hemoglobin species occurring in adults. Carriers of β-thalassemia are mostly found in the Mediterranean countries, whereas carriers of α-thalassemia are mostly found in Southeast Asia.

The term α-thalassemia refers to hemoglobinopathies in which there is reduced synthesis of the α-chains. Since α-chains are contained in fetal Hb (HbF) as well as in HbA_0 and HBA_2, α-chain thalassemia has an impact on the fetus and patients of all ages. The absence of the α-chains is offset in the fetus by the formation of tetramers of γ-chains ($Hb\gamma_4$ = Bart's Hb), after birth by the formation of tetramers of β-chains ($Hb\beta_4$ = HbH). Erythrocytes containing these pathologic hemoglobins have a tendency to aggregate, however, and are broken down early. Since the synthesis of α-chains is coded for by 2 genes with 4 alleles, 4 clinical pictures of varying severity can be identified, depending on the number of defective genes: a defect in one gene is manifested merely as an increased proportion of the above-mentioned pathologic variants of hemoglobin, a 2-allele defect produces mild (α-thalassemia minor), a 3-allele defect pronounced anemia with premature hemolysis (HbH disease). The complete loss of the α-chains is incompatible with the survival of the fetus.

In contrast to α-thalassemia, β-thalassemia does not have an effect until infancy or childhood when the γ-chains are replaced by β-chains. If this is not possible, HbF (with γ-chains) and HbA_2 (with δ-chains) are formed by way of compensation. Depending on its mode of inheritance, a distinction can be made between a heterozygous form (thalassemia minor) with reduced β-chain synthesis and correspondingly milder anemia, and a homozygous form (thalassemia major) with more or less complete absence of β-chains and severe anemia.

The pathologic variants of hemoglobin in thalassemia lead to characteristic abnormalities in the shape of erythrocytes (microcytic anemia with target cells, Fig. 18), which are detectable microscopically. More precise differentiation is possible by hemoglobin electrophoresis or PCR.

Pathophysiologically, these structural and morphologic abnormalities of erythrocytes result in more or less pronounced insufficiency as oxygen carriers and lead to an increased aggregation tendency. In addition, deformation also leads to accelerated destruction of erythrocytes, predominantly in the spleen, with all the signs of corpuscular hemolytic anemia. For signs of hemolysis and hemolytically determined iron overload, *see under "Pathologically Increased Hemolysis"*.

Due to immigration from the Mediterranean area β-thalassemia is today also a challenge for the differenital diagnosis of microcytic anemias in the countries of Central and Northern Europe. In hypochromic microcytic anemia, thalassemia is the most important differential diagnosis of iron deficiency. At the same time, the erythrocyte count is mostly normal or even elevated, the concentration of sTfR is high. The resulting inadequately increased iron resorption leads, together with possibly required blood transfusions, to iron overload.

Disturbances of Porphyrin Synthesis

Disturbances of porphyrin synthesis [23] are to be considered here only in so far as they may affect erythropoiesis and lead to anemia (Fig. 19).

These forms of anemia are called siderochrestic, since the iron provided for Hb synthesis in the bone marrow cannot be used, despite adequate reserves, and is consequently stored in the erythroblasts. The erythroblasts, which are thus overloaded with iron, are then termed sideroblasts. They can be detected in the bone marrow using iron-specific stains. In sideroachrestic anemia, however, the inadequately increased iron absorption results in the development of generalized, genuine iron overload over a longer period. Especially after repeated transfusions, it is

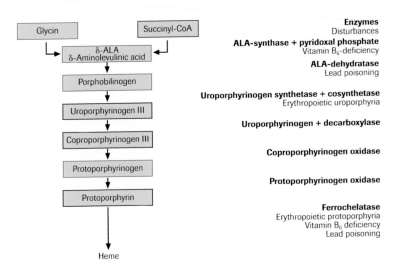

Fig. 19: Disturbances of porphyrin synthesis with possible anemia

recognizable from an elevated serum ferritin concentration. Most of the causes of sideroachrestic anemia are comparatively uncommon, and therefore rarely need to be considered in practice. Hereditary erythropoietic porphyrias such as congenital erythropoietic uroporphyria (Günther's disease) with a defect of uroporphyrinogen III-synthase and erythropoietic protoporphyria with a defect of ferrochelatase are particularly rare. Acquired forms such as pyridoxal phosphate (vitamin B_6) deficiency are slightly more common. This may be of nutritional origin, in alcoholics, for example, or arise as a result of isoniazid therapy in tuberculosis patients, and leads to a disturbance of iron incorporation via inhibition of δ-amino-levulinic acid synthase and ferrochelatase. Similar pathologic mechanisms are also at the root of lead-induced anemia and disturbance of porphyrin synthesis. Chronic lead intoxication leads to inhibition of δ-amino-levulinic acid dehydratase and of ferrochelatase. All the above-mentioned causes ultimately produce a disturbance of iron utilization via the synthesis of an incomplete porphyrin skeleton or via the direct inhibition of ferrochelatase, with the general features of sideroachrestic (sideroblastic) anemia described above. If the defect is mainly in the terminal stage of the reaction (incorporation of iron by ferrochelatase), zinc is incorporated into the finished protoporphyrin skeleton instead of iron, recognizable from the increased concentration of Zn-protoporphyrin in the erythrocytes. Defects at earlier stages in porphyrin synthesis can be identified by the analysis of the corresponding intermediate products; lead and vitamin B_6 can also be determined directly for confirmation of the diagnosis.

Pathologically Increased Hemolysis

"Hemolysis" is the term generally used in clinical medicine to describe the pathologically increased destruction of erythrocytes. The cause of this may lie in structural or biochemical defects in the erythrocytes themselves ("corpuscular hemolysis"), in which case it takes place mainly in the macrophages of the RES in the spleen or the liver. By contrast, extracorpuscular hemolysis takes place mainly intravascularly through the action of autoantibodies, toxins, infective organisms or physical noxae, such as artificial heart valves. Intravascular hemolysis can be detected very sensitively by means of clinico-chemical investigations, since hemoglobin and erythrocyte enzymes, e.g. LDH isoenzymes 1 and 2, pass into the peripheral blood even at a low hemolysis rate.

Haptoglobin

Since free hemoglobin is rapidly bound to α_2-haptoglobin and this hemoglobin–haptoglobin complex is also rapidly phagocytized by the RES, a selective reduction in free haptoglobin is regarded as the most sensitive sign of intravascular hemolysis which at the same time also has a high degree of diagnostic specificity. The only other possible causes are severe protein-loss syndromes or disturbances of protein synthesis. This applies in particular to advanced liver diseases (e.g., liver cirrhosis) with a severe synthesis defect which also includes haptoglobin. A reduction in haptoglobin may also be produced, albeit less commonly, by gastrointestinal protein-loss syndromes which also non-selectively include macromolecular proteins, such as celiac disease, Whipple's disease. Since haptoglobin also serves as a proteinase inhibitor, its synthesis in the liver is increased during acute-phase reactions. The resultant increase in concentration may then "mask" any hemolysis which is present simultaneously (Table 5).

Table 5: Differentiation: hemolysis, acute-phase reaction, and protein loss or disturbance of protein synthesis

Disease	Haptoglobin	Hemopexin	CRP
Mild hemolysis	↓–↓↓	n	n
Severe hemolysis	↓↓	↓	n
Hemolysis and acute-phase reaction	n–↑	n–↓	↑↑
Acute-phase reaction	↑–↑↑	n	↑↑
Nephrotic syndrome	↑–↑↑	↓	n–↓
Gastrointestinal protein loss or disturbance of protein synthesis	↓	↓	n–↓

Features of Severe Hemolysis

Free hemoglobin occurs in the plasma only if the hemoglobin-binding capacity of haptpoglobin is exceeded. If the renal threshold is exceeded, hemoglobin excretion in the urine may also occur. Excess heme can also be bound by hemopexin and be removed from the plasma in the form of a heme-hemopexin complex. Hemoglobinuria and a reduction in serum hemopexin concentration are thus signs of severe hemolysis.

The degradation of heme leads, independently of the site of the hemolytic process, to an increased concentration of unconjugated bilirubin and of iron. Because of the simultaneous inappropriately increased iron absorption and the possible need for transfusions, all chronic forms of hemolysis are associated with iron overload, recognizable as an increased serum ferritin concentration. With adequate bone marrow function, increased hemolysis, especially extracorpuscular forms, can be compensated for by enhanced erythropoiesis which can be boosted up to 10-fold. This is shown as an increased passage of immature erythrocytes (reticulocytes) into the peripheral blood. Anemia, which may be macrocytic (due to the increased volume of the reticulocytes), develops only if the hemolysis rate exceeds the bone marrow capacity for erythropoiesis.

If, in the long run, the binding capacity of haptoglobin and hemopexin is exceeded during severe intravascular hemolysis and as a consequence of this, larger amounts of free hemoglobin are filtered through the glomeruli and therefore excreted, then in individual cases because of the chronic loss of iron, the hemolysis may lead to iron deficiency. If, however, iron loss does not occur in this manner, then iron overload is usually the consequence of chronic hemolysis as described above. This can be differentiated by regular urine investigations and ferritin determinations in serum.

Causes of Hemolysis (Corpuscular/Extracorpuscular)

Corpuscular hemolysis can be induced by defects in the erythrocyte membrane, in addition to the hemoglobinopathies such as sickle-cell anemia or thalassemia as mentioned earlier. The most important example of such a membrane defect is spherocytic anemia (hereditary spherocytosis) which can be diagnosed on the basis of the characteristic morphologic changes ("spherocytes") (Table 6) and the reduced osmotic resistance of the erythrocytes. Other causes are defects of erythrocyte enzymes, e.g. glucose-6-phosphatedehydrogenase deficiency, which are required for the stabilization of functionally important proteins. This

Fundamentals

Table 6: Diagnosis of corpuscular hemolytic anemias

Disease	Erythrocyte Forms	Confirmation Test
Hereditary spherocytosis	Microspherocytes	Osmotic Resistance
Thalassemia	Target cells	Hemoglobin electrophoresis, PCR
Sickle cell anemia	Sickle cells	Hemoglobin electrophoresis, PCR
Erythrocyte enzyme defects (e.g. glucose-6-phosphate dehydrogenase-deficiency)	unspecific Heinz Bodies	Erythrocyte enzymes
PNH (paroxysmal nocturnal hemoglobinuria or Machiafava-Micheli syndrome), defect of glycolipid FACS (Fluorescence Activated Cell Sorting) anchor antigens (CD59, CD55)	unspecific	

disease not only is most frequently observed in individuals of African and Mediterranean origin, but has also become important in Central and Northern Europe as a result of immigration. The most important acquired corpuscular form of hemolysis is represented by PNH (Paroxysmal Nocturnal Hemoglobinuria) (Table 6). All other defects of erythrocyte enzymes are definitely rarities.

Numerous noxae, most of which can be identified from the case history or by means of simple laboratory investigations, produce intravascular hemolysis by directly damaging the erythrocytes themselves. These include mechanical hemolysis after heart valve replacement, toxins such as snake venoms or detergents, and infective organisms such as malarial plasmodia, or hemolysis as a consequence of gram-negative sepsis. Intravascular hemolysis can be identified independently of the causes on the basis of the above-mentioned general features of hemolysis. However, in the case of the autoimmune hemolytic anemias which can occur in the context of autoimmune diseases, immune defects, viral infections, lymphatic malignancies, and as drug-induced anemias, the causes are often difficult to determine in the individual case. A distinction is made between so-called warm, cold, and bithermal (Donath-Landsteiner) antibodies. Binding of the antibodies to the patient's erythrocytes can be detected in the direct anti-human globulin test (Coombs' test). If the result is positive, further differentiation using other methods is necessary.

Diagnosis of Disturbances
of Iron Metabolism

Iron Balance

Disturbances of iron metabolism are mainly due to disturbances in iron balance which, in turn, are mainly due to disturbances in the resorption of iron or iron losses. Therefore, the uptake of iron occupies the key position in the iron metabolism as a whole.

The daily iron requirement depends on age and sex. It is increased in puberty and in pregnancy. Under physiologic conditions, the total iron pool is more or less constant in adults. The quantity of iron absorbed is about 10% (1 mg) of the quantity consumed daily in the normal diet, but this fraction can increase from 20 to 40% (2–4 mg) in conditions of iron deficiency.

Physiologic loss of iron is low, and comparable to the quantity absorbed. It takes place as a result of the shedding of intestinal epithelial cells and through excretion in bile, urine, and perspiration. Since the absorption and the loss of iron are limited under physiologic conditions, the quantity of storage iron can only be increased by massive supplies from outside the body. Thus, every transfusion of one liter of blood increases the quantity of storage iron in the body by about 250 mg.

Disturbances in iron absorption can be detected by an iron absorption test. After collecting a blood sample from a fasting patient to determine the baseline value for the serum iron concentration, approximately 200 mg of a bivalent iron preparation is administered. A second blood collection is performed after 3 hours. With normal iron absorption, there should be an increase to 2–3 times the baseline value during the observation period.

A reduced or delayed rise indicates a disturbance of iron absorption. An increased rise is found in rare forms of iron deficiency, and in primary hemochromatosis [88].

The excess of iron that is not used for the synthesis of hemoglobin, myoglobin, or iron enzymes is stored in the depot proteins ferritin and hemosiderin.

The total iron content of the healthy human body is about 3.5–4 g in women and 4–5 g in men [66]. About 70% of this is stored in hemoglobin, 10% is contained in myoglobin and iron-containing and, 20% in the

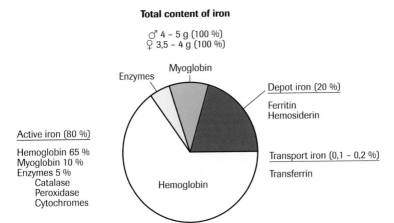

Fig. 20: Total content of iron in the body

body's iron depot, and only 0.1 to 0.2% is bound to transferrin as transport iron. However, this distribution applies only under optimum nutritional conditions (Fig. 20).

---

1 g of hemoglobin is equal to 3.4 mg of iron

Since the life cycle of the red blood cells is 120 days, an adult requires about 16–20 mg of iron daily in order to replace these vital cells [25]. Most of the iron required for this purpose comes from lysed red blood cells.

During pregnancy, birth, and breast-feeding, the additional iron requirement is far in excess of the quantity of absorbable iron contained in the food. The loss of iron in normal menstruation is about 15–30 mg (100 mL of blood contains about 50 mg of iron). The additional iron requirement during pregnancy is between 700 and 1000 mg.

As a result of menstruation and pregnancy, the quantity of depot iron in women decreases through blood loss to 250 mg, i.e. only 5–10% of the total iron content. According to a WHO estimate, 50% of all fertile women in western countries suffer from hypoferremia.

The second largest component in active iron is the muscular myoglobin, at about 10%. Like hemoglobin, myoglobin is an oxygen-binding hemoprotein with a molecular weight of about 17,100 D. Because it has a higher affinity for oxygen than hemoglobin, myoglobin is responsible for the uptake and storage of oxygen in the muscle cells.

The diagnostic specificity of the serum myoglobin determination is limited, since it is not possible to differentiate between skeletal muscle myoglobin and myocardium myoglobin. An increase in the serum is observed in all forms of muscle disease and injuries, and in myocardial infarction. The diagnostic value in the assessment of impaired kidney function is limited, since myoglobin is completely eliminated with the urine or reabsorbed. The determination of myoglobin in sports medicine for the assessment of performance is worthy of mention.

Case History and Clinical Findings

Ferritin, Transferrin, Transferrin Saturation, Soluble Transferrin Receptor

According to WHO criteria (World Health Organization. Nutritional anemias. Series 1992: 503), anemia exists when the concentration of hemoglobin falls below the values listed in Table 7.

Table 7: Criteria for anemia

Adults	Hb [g/dL]
Men	13.5
Women (<50 yr)	12.5
Women (>50 yr)	13.5
Children (<16 yr)	11.5

Anemia may be caused by:
- Deficiency of iron, vitamin B_{12}, vitamin B_6, folate
- Chronic disturbances of iron distribution, chronic inflammation
- Anemias of infection
- Tumor anemias
- Chronic disturbances of utilization, uremic anemias
- Blood loss
- Erythrocytic decomposition (hemolysis)
- Impaired erythrocyte formation (toxic or neoplastic processes)
- Genetic defects

Table 8: Case history and clinical findings in patients with anemia

Case history	• Hemolytic disturbances of genetic origin. • Dizziness, shortness of breath, paleness, icterus. • Unusual stools. • History of gynecological bleeding. • Eating and drinking habits (iron deficiency in vegetarians, vitamin B_{12} deficiency, and alcoholism). • Hemolysis and aplasia induced by medication.
Clinical findings	• Advanced anemia: Fatigue, shortness of breath, and dizziness. • Additional iron deficiency: Angular stomatitis, brittle nails, and brittle hair. • Hemolysis: Flu-like symptoms with discoloration of sclera, skin and urine, occasional splenodynia, ostalgia. • Vitamin B_{12} deficiency: Subicteric colorite, inflammation of the tongue, occasional signs of bleeding combined with thrombocytopenia, occasional paresthesia. • Macrocytic anemias in patients with chronic liver disease (alcohol-related and non-alcohol-related).

The following laboratory parameters in particular have become significant and enjoy widespread application:

Biochemical parameters: Ferritin (iron deficiency), transferrin, transferrin saturation (iron overload), soluble transferrin receptor (disturbances of iron distribution and utilization), C-reactive protein (inflammations), ceruloplasmin (iron redistribution), haptoglobin (increased iron turnover), vitamin B_6, and vitamin B_{12}, folate (deficiencies).

Hematologic parameters: Hemoglobin, hematocrit, red blood cell count, reticulocyte count, mean cellular hemoglobin content of reticulocytes (Ret-Hb), reticulocyte production index (RPI).

Ferritin is the most important iron storage protein. Together with the quantitatively and biologically less important hemosiderin, it contains about 15–20% of all the iron in the body. Ferritin occurs in nearly all organs. Particularly high concentrations are found in the liver, spleen, and bone marrow.

Clinical Aspects

A direct correlation is found for healthy adults between the plasma ferritin concentration and the quantity of available iron stored in the body. Comparative studies with quantitative phlebotomies and the histochemical assessment of bone marrow aspirates have shown that in iron deficiency and in primary or secondary stages of iron overload ferritin provides accurate information on the iron reserves available to the body for hemoglobin synthesis.

If more iron is supplied than the body can store as ferritin, iron is deposited as hemosiderin in the cells of the reticuloendothelial system. Unlike ferritin, hemosiderin is insoluble in water, and it is only with difficulty that its iron content can be mobilized.

Table 9: Limits of ferritin determination in the assessment of iron deficiency

- Indirect information only regarding the supply of erythropoiesis with iron
- No real-time indication of the severity of iron deficiency in the case of low or borderline low serum ferritin values, especially in young children, adolescents in a growth spurt, serious athletes, blood donors, pregnant women
- Disproportional increase with:
  - Infections, acute, and chronic inflammation, malignant tumors
  - Damage of the liver parenchyma, by e.g., viral or alcoholic acute or chronic hepatitis, liver cirrhosis
  - Dialysis patients
  - Myelodisplastic syndrome (MDS)
  - Parenteral iron administration

Table 10: Merits of the various parameters for the detection of iron deficiency

Parameter	Sensitivity (%)	Specificity (%)	Efficiency (%)
Serum iron +	84	43	52
Transferrin	84	63	67
Serum ferritin	79	96	92
Serum iron + Serum ferritin	84	42	51
Transferrin + Serum ferritin	84	50	64
Soluble transferrin receptor/ferritin index	92	84	

Ferritin is synthesized in the cells in response to the intracellular iron concentration. If the intracellular iron is high, the synthesis of ferritin is increased. If the intracellular iron concentration is low, the synthesis of ferritin is downregulated. A small amount of the ferritin produced is secreted by the cells into the bloodstream. A direct correlation between the amount of stored iron and serum ferritin exists when the serum ferritin concentration is in the range from 12 to 200 µg/L.

> **1 µg/L (ng/mL) serum ferritin corresponds to 10 mg stored iron**

Serum ferritin is a good indicator of storage iron reserves, but it provides no information about the functional compartment, for instance the amount of iron actually available for erythropoiesis. A low serum ferritin value merely indicates that the patient is at risk of developing active iron deficiency. In patients with infections, acute chronic inflammation and malignant tumors normal or elevated serum ferritin values can occur, despite active iron deficiency. The result is a disproportional increase in serum ferritin in relation to the storage iron reserves. In patients with ferritin values in the reference range accompanied by elevated C-reactive protein values (CRP is an indicator of an acute-phase reaction) a storage iron deficiency cannot be ruled out. Diseases and conditions in which the serum ferritin level does not reflect the content of storage iron are listed in Table 11.

Table 11: Clinical significance of ferritin determination

---

1. Representative result

Detection of prelatent and latent iron deficiency
Differential diagnosis of anemias
Monitoring of high-risk groups
Monitoring of iron therapy (oral)
Determination of the iron status of dialysis patients and patients who have received
    multiple blood transfusions
Diagnosis of iron overload
Monitoring of phlebotomy therapy or chelating agent therapy

---

2. Non-representative result

Destruction of hepatocellular tissue
Infections
Inflammations (collagen diseases)
Malignancies
Iron therapy (parenteral)

Clinical Aspects

The value of ferritin determination was demonstrated in a comparison of the various parameters available for the determination of the body's iron stores [101].

Ferritin is well suited for assessment of the iron metabolism of a patient population having no primary consumptive disease or chronic inflammation. The determination of ferritin is particularly useful in the diagnosis of disturbances of iron metabolism, in the monitoring of iron therapy, for the determination of iron reserves in high-risk groups, and in the differential diagnosis of anemias (Table 11).

In clinical practice, the ferritin concentration reflects the size of the iron stores, especially at the beginning of therapy. A deficiency in the stores of the reticuloendothelial system (RES) can be detected at a particularly early stage. A value of 20 ng/mL has been found to be a suitable clinical limit for prelatent iron deficiency. A value below this reliably indicates exhaustion of the iron reserves that can be mobilized for hemoglobin synthesis. A decrease to less than 12 ng/mL has been defined as latent iron deficiency. Neither of these values calls for further laboratory confirmation, even where the blood count is still normal. They are indications for therapy, though it is still necessary to look for the cause of the iron deficiency. If the reduced ferritin concentration is accompanied by hypochromic microcytic anemia, the patient is suffering from manifest iron deficiency (Table 12).

If the ferritin level is elevated and a disturbance of distribution can be ruled out by determination of the transferrin saturation and/or of the C-reactive protein and by investigation of the blood sedimentation rate and the blood count, the raised ferritin level indicates that the body is overloaded with iron. A ferritin value of 400 ng/mL is taken as a limit. The transferrin saturation is massively increased (over 45%) in these cases.

If there is no evidence of any other disease, primary or secondary hemochromatosis must be suspected. Differential diagnosis must be pursued through history-taking, genetic analysis, liver biopsy, bone-

Table 12: Ferritin concentrations in patients with iron deficiency and iron overload [67]

Prelatent iron deficiency (storage iron deficiency)	<20 ng/mL
Latent iron deficiency/iron deficiency anemia	<12 ng/mL
Representative iron overload	>400 ng/mL

Clinical Aspects

marrow puncture, or magnetic resonance imaging (MRI). Diagnosis of a primary hemochromatosis calls for further investigations for organic lesions and genetic testing.

Raised ferritin values are ambiguous, and are found in a number of inflammatory diseases, in the presence of malignant growths, and in the presence of damage to the liver parenchyma. Elevated ferritin levels are also found in a number of anemias arising from various causes in some cases with true iron overload. Recent oral or, in particular, parenteral iron therapy can also lead to raised non-representative ferritin values.

The increases in the ferritin concentration are frequently due to disturbances of distribution, and differential diagnosis is possible by determination of transferrin concentration and of transferrin saturation. In all these processes, the transferrin value is reduced or close to the lower limit of the reference range (<200 mg/dL). The transferrin saturation is low to normal (<15%), and hypochromic anemia can often be diagnosed on the basis of the blood cell count.

In healthy individuals, 15–45% of the transferrin is saturated with iron. When the supply of the functional iron compartment is inadequate, transferrin synthesis is increased by way of compensation, which leads to a decrease in the transferrin saturation. In the presence of infec-

Clinical Aspects

Table 13: Transferrin in the differential diagnosis of disturbances of iron metabolism

1. Normal to slightly reduced transferrin concentrations
Primary hemochromatosis-exception: late stage secondary hemochromatosis

2. Decreased transferrin concentrations
Infections Inflammations/collagen diseases Malignant tumors Hemodialysis patients Cirrhosis of the liver-disturbances of synthesis Nephrotic syndrome Ineffective erythropoiesis (e.g. sideroachrestic and megaloblastic anemias) Thalassemias

3. Increased transferrin concentrations
Iron deficiency Estrogen-induced increase in transferrin synthesis (pregnancy, medication) Ineffective erythropoiesis in some cases (e.g. myelodysplastic syndromes)

tions, acute or chronic inflammation, and malignant tumors, transferrin synthesis is downregulated regardless of the status of active iron. For this reason, transferrin saturation is not an indicator of supply of the functional iron compartment and cannot be used in any anemia accompanied by an increase in C-reactive protein. Conditions and diseases in which the transferrin saturation does not provide relevant results for diagnosing iron deficiency are listed in Table 14.

Table 14: Disadvantages of the determination of transferrin saturation for assessing iron deficiency

- Transferrin is an anti-acute-phase protein, its synthesis is reduced in the presence of infections, inflammation, and malignant tumors regardless of iron supply.
- Transferrin is released in the presence of acute hepatocellular damage, resulting in serum transferrin concentration that is inadequately high.
- Pregnancy and estrogen therapy lead to an increase in transferrin synthesis, independent of iron supply.
- Transferrin saturation is increased for hours after a meal.
- Transferrin saturation does not drop below 15% until the iron stores are empty and Hb is 2 g/dL below its baseline value.

Elevated transferrin values are found in the presence of iron deficiency and particularly in pregnancy. The transferrin level may also be raised as a result of drug induction (administration of oral contraceptives). A detailed patient history is essential.

A number of rare anemias with hyperferritinemia and low transferrin levels belong to the group of sideroachrestic diseases and may be congenital hypochromic microcytic anemias (atransferrinemia, auto-transferrin antibodies, receptor defects, and porphyrias).

Increased ferritin concentrations together with low transferrin levels may also point to anemias with ineffective erythropoiesis (thalassemias, megaloblastic, sideroblastic, and dyserythropoietic anemias). Myelodysplastic syndromes, on the other hand, may initially be accompanied by elevated values for both transferrin and ferritin.

Elevated ferritin concentrations unrelated to the iron stores are often found in patients with malignancies. Possible reasons that have been suggested for this phenomenon are increased ferritin synthesis by neoplastic cells, release of ferritin on decomposition of neoplastic tissue, and blockage of erythropoiesis as a result of chronic inflammatory processes in and around the tumor tissue. Ferritin determinations on patients with malignant tumors sometimes also record high concentrations of acidic isoferritins.

In the presence of inflammations, infectious diseases, or malignant tumors, low transferrin concentrations and low transferrin saturation values point to disturbances of iron distribution. Low transferrin concentrations may be caused either by losses (renal and intestinal) or by reduced synthesis (compensation and liver damage).

Low transferrin values found for patients with cirrhosis of the liver are usually due to the defective protein metabolism. In nephrotic syndrome, so much transferrin is lost via the urine that low transferrin levels are the rule. The excretion of transferrin in the urine is also used to determine the selectivity of proteinuria.

The transferrin concentration and the transferrin saturation are valuable aids in the differential diagnosis of raised ferritin concentrations. True iron overload is accompanied by increased transferrin saturation. Non-representative ferritin elevation in patients with disturbances of distribution is characterized by low transferrin saturation and low transferrin concentrations.

Soluble transferrin receptor (sTfR) arises from proteolysis of the intact protein on the cell surface, leading to monomers that can be measured in plasma and serum. The concentration of sTfR behaves proportionally to the number of intact TfR molecules on the plasma membrane of the cells. Thus, the concentration of sTfR in plasma or serum is an indirect measure of total TfR and reflects either the cellular need for iron or the rate of erythropoiesis.

Measurement of sTfR is used to diagnose iron deficiency in individuals with chronic disease (inflammatory diseases, infections, and malignancies); many of them are anemic. Furthermore, the determination of sTfR is a valuable supplement to the determination of ferritin in individuals known to have limited storage iron, e.g. young children, adolescents in a growth spurt, serious athletes, blood donors, and pregnants.

The level of sTfR is a summation of the TfR portion regulated by the intracellular iron concentration and a portion correlated to the amount of erythropoietic cells. Since the latter may be reduced in the presence of tumor anemias and anemias of chronic inflammations the upper reference range value of sTfR is not reached in about 50% of these cases, despite functional iron deficiency.

Clinical Aspects

Iron deficiency, regardless of the cause, leads to an increased expression of the transferrin receptor and, accordingly, to an increased concentration of the sTfR. All forms of marked storage iron deficiency can be detected with a great deal of certainty by a low plasma ferritin concentration. Measuring of sTfR therefore does not offer an advantage in these cases. In cases with adequate iron reserves coupled with functional iron deficiency, i.e., disturbances of iron utilization, an increased concentration of sTfR indicates inadequate supply of iron to erythropoiesis or inadequate iron mobilization [142].

Patients with malignant neoplasias and chronic inflammation develop a deficiency of transport and active iron accompanied by a simultaneous relative overloading of the iron stores and a simultaneous relative inadequate supply of iron to the erythropoietic cells (as a consequence of reduced transferrin synthesis, among other things). The reduced availability of iron is a protective mechanism as well as one of the major pathomechanisms in anemia of chronic disease (ACD). When the disturbance of iron distribution is pronounced, the presence of a hypochromic anemia can be assumed. It can be distinguished from iron deficiency anemia by ferritin determination. In addition to reduced transferrin synthesis, an increased release of cytokines such as IFN-γ and TNF-α leads to an increased iron uptake in macrophages by means of an increased transferrin receptor expression. In the presence of ACD and tumors, this increased iron storage in macrophages also withdraws a portion of the iron from transferrin, which is already reduced. A further cause for the development of anemia is the reduced erythropoietic activity. This is definitively not due to an erythropoietin deficiency but rather a possible disturbed regulation induced by cytokines. In the majority of cases of disturbed iron distribution, an inadequate supply of iron to the erythropoietic cells coupled with a reduced erythropoietic activity is present. Accordingly, the transferrin receptor expression is usually normal.

Disturbances of iron utilization and incorporation that simulate the clinical picture of an iron deficiency anemia are also possible in the presence of normal iron reserves and normal iron distribution indicated by the presence of a normal ferritin concentration since they can also lead to a microcytic anemia. Since erythropoietin administration has replaced formerly common transfusions used to treat anemias, dialysis patients now represent the largest group of individuals with this type of anemia [61, 130].

The ferritin concentration is generally a true reflection of the iron reserves (an exception to this is when it is immediately preceded by iron replacement or in the presence of a secondary disorder involving iron distribution disturbances) and can therefore be used as a guideline for recognizing any depot iron deficiency or for avoiding iron overload in iron replacement therapy. Transferrin saturation is currently the best indicator of the presence of mobilized transport iron and is inversely proportional to the iron requirement. Reduced transferrin saturation in dialysis patients is a sign of inadequate iron mobilization and therefore of a functional iron deficiency requiring iron replacement. It is possible to use the concentration of sTfR as direct indicator of the iron requirement. On no account can the sTfR replace the ferritin determination for assessing the iron reserves as it only reflects the current erythropoietic activity and/or its iron requirement, which does not necessarily correlate with the iron reserves.

All iron overload states can be detected using clinical chemistry methods based on the elevated plasma ferritin concentration, the simultaneously elevated iron level and the increased transferrin saturation in the presence of transferrin synthesis that is usually reduced by way of compensation. Depending on the cause of iron overload, the transferrin receptor expression can be very different depending on whether the erythropoiesis is increased or reduced. Accordingly, an elevated concentration of the sTfR is also found in the presence of all hemolytic states with an erythropoietic activity that is increased by way of compensation. In patients with renal insufficiency (without erythropoietin therapy), a reduced transferrin receptor expression corresponding to a greatly reduced erythropoiesis is found. Erythropoiesis is not immediately affected in the presence of hematochromatosis. Transferrin receptor expression can be normal or reduced [10, 38].

Laboratory Diagnostics of Suspected Disturbances of Iron Metabolism

The following steps are recommended in the diagnosis of disturbances or iron metabolism ([139], Fig. 21):

- Blood count to identify an anemia. An anemia exists when the hemoglobin concentration falls below the following values [67]:

Females	12.3 g/dL
Males	14.0 g/dL

- Ferritin in the serum to assess the storage iron reserves. An iron deficiency exists and oral iron replacement is indicated when the serum ferritin values fall below the following values [67]:

Females	13 µg/L
Males	30 µg/L

- Serum CRP to determine if an inflammatory reaction influences the ferritin value.

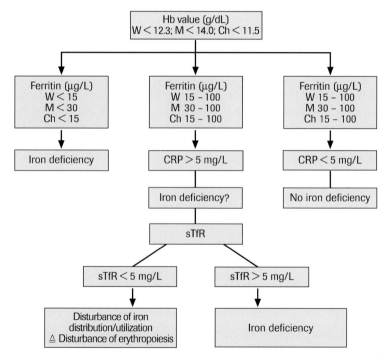

Fig. 21: Successive diagnostics in cases of suspected disturbances of iron metabolism (W = women, M = men, Ch = children)

Clinical Aspects

- Relevant iron deficiency is not present if CRP is ≤5 mg/L with ferritin values of 15–150 µg/L in women, and in the presence of ferritin values of 30–400 µg/L in men. If the CRP level exceeds 5 mg/L, the ferritin value can be inadequately high in relation to the storage iron reserves. In this case, ferritin values in the range of 15 (30)–150 (400) µg/L provide no conclusive information about iron supply.
- sTfR in serum to assess the iron supply of erythropoiesis.
  - If the concentration is normal, assessment may not be possible, because the sTfR concentration can be in the reference range in the presence of ACD and tumor anemia due to hypoproliferative erythropoiesis, despite a functional iron deficiency.
  - If the sTfR concentration is elevated, the iron supply of erythropoiesis is inadequate if the corrected reticulocyte index is normal or low. An elevated sTfR value indicates the presence of an inadequate iron supply.
- Hemoglobin content of the reticulocytes (Ret-Hb).

An increase in Ret-Hb of >2 pg or a permanent Ret-Hb >28 pg is an indicator of an adequate amount of iron entering the red cell precursors; a Ret-Hb < 28 pg may indicate functional ID.

Using the Ret-Hb to define hypochromic erythropoiesis, the cut-off values for ferritin, sTfR, and sTfR/log ferritin (ferritin index) in patients

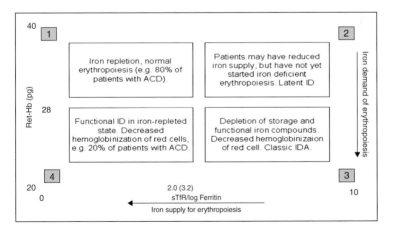

Fig. 22: Plot for identifying the different erythropoietic states of advancing ID [139]

with and without acute-phase response (based on a CRP cut-off of 5 mg/L) can be assessed. Functional ID is defined as a Ret-Hb < 28 pg, based on the distribution of these values in healthy controls. The biochemical markers performed significantly better in the absence of inflammation: the cut-off for the ferritin index is 3.2 for ID without acute phase reaction (APR; CRP ≤ 5 mg/L) and 2.0 for ID combined with anemia of chronic disease (ACD), anemia of infection, chronic inflammation, end-stage renal failure, and cancer-related anemia. In anemia, the relationship between Ret-Hb and the ferritin index can be depicted by a simple plot (Fig. 22).

Four quadrants can be identified based on the respective cut-off values for Ret-Hb and the ferritin index. The quadrants shown in these plots correspond to different hypo- or normoregenerative erythropoietic states:

1. Normochromic erythropoiesis with repleted iron stores (iron status in ACD).
2. Normochromic erythropoiesis with depleted iron stores but not yet in an iron-deficient erythropoietic state (latent iron deficiency).
3. Hypoproliferative erythropoiesis, depletion of storage and functional iron compounds (classic iron deficiency), decreased hemoglobinization of red cells.
4. Hypoproliferative erythropoiesis, functional ID in iron-repleted stores (functional ID in patients with ACD), decreased hemoglobinization of red cells.

The following limitations should be considered in order to effectively use the plot:

1. An increase of erythroid precursor cell mass (hemolytic syndrome, myelodysplastic syndrome, and pregnancy) may shift data points from quadrant 1 to quadrant 2. This is caused by an increase in sTfR which correlates with erythroid precursor mass.
2. Patients with β-thalassemia trait may have data points in quadrant 4 even though they do not have functional iron deficiency.
3. Iron-supplemented patients with ACD may have data points in quadrant 2 or 3, but near the ferritin index cut-off. In these cases the iron supplementation may increase erythrocyte maturation and elevate sTfR, mostly within the reference range.
4. In cancer patients with chemotherapy-induced anemia and hypochromic cells, Ret-Hb may have inadequately high values.

5. A low reticulocyte count may cause large variations in the calculation of Ret-Hb as hematology analyzers only measure fixed red cell counts (sum of erythrocytes and reticulocytes) in the sample.
6. The 95% confidence intervals for Ret-Hb of 28 pg and ferritin indices of 3.2 and 2.0 are 27–29 pg, 3.0–3.4 and 1.9–2.1, respectively. Samples with data points in quadrants 2 and 3 but within the confidence intervals of the ferritin index should be assessed clinically as belonging to erythropoietic status 1 and 4, respectively.
7. Other deficiency states than ID may also cause low Ret-Hb. So, Ret-HB <28 pg is no definite proof of ID.

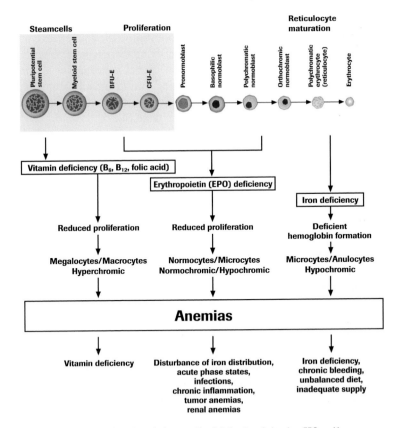

Fig. 23: Disturbances of erythropoiesis caused by deficiencies of vitamins, EPO, and iron

Most Frequent Disturbances of Iron Metabolism and Erythropoiesis

Erythropoietin (EPO) is the most important growth factor for the regulation of erythropoiesis. Additionally, erythropoiesis is controlled primarily by iron (Fig. 23).

Hypochromic, Microcytic Anemias

The most frequently occurring iron metabolism anemias are iron deficiency and disturbances of iron distribution. They are hypochromic anemias and are often microcytic or normocytic. Medical practices currently dedicate significant resources to clarifying these types of anemia. In addition to iron deficiency, which is widespread, disturbances of iron distribution caused by tumors, infections or chronic inflammations are increasing markedly. A very clear classification of anemias has been used in hematologic diagnostics for years (Table 15).

Table 15: Classification of anemias based on erythrocyte indices (MCH, MCV) and reticulocyte count

MCH (pg/cell)	hypochromic <28	normochromic 28–33	hyperchromic >33
MCV (fL)	microcytic <80	normocytic 80–96	macrocytic >96
Reticulocyte production index	hyporegenerative <2	normoregenerative 2	hyperregenerative >2

MCH = Hemoglobin content of erythrocytes (mean cellular hemoglobin)
MCV = Mean cellular volume of erythrocytes

MCH and MCV are automatically determined by all modern cell instruments. Their determination is indispensable to the classification of hypochromic anemias (Fig. 24).

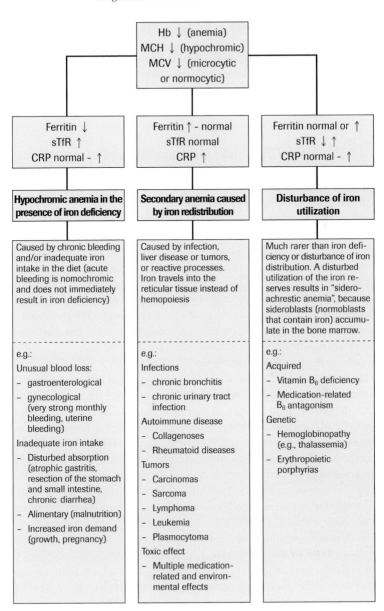

Fig. 24: Diagnosis of hypochromic anemias

Iron Deficiency – Diagnosis and Therapy

In the case of a negative iron balance, the iron stores are reduced first; this can be seen from the measurement of ferritin. The concentration of active iron decreases only at a relatively late stage (as shown by the lower transferrin saturation or the higher sTfR concentration).

Laboratory Diagnostis of Suspected Iron Deficiency

Diagnosis of non-manifest iron deficiency is practically impossible by clinical methods. The subjective condition of patients with iron deficiency does not reveal any definitely attributable changes. The familiar clinical symptoms such as pallor, weakness, loss of concentration, exertional dyspnea, and reduced resistance to infection appear only with the development of active iron anemia. The relatively specific changes in the skin and mucous membranes, atrophic glossitis and gastritis, cracks at the corners of the mouth, and atrophy of the hair and nails are late symptoms. An important observation is that iron deficiency often accompanies serious, life-threatening conditions, and can therefore serve as an indicator of such diseases in case of blood loss.

According to the literature, up to 5% of children and adolescents, 10% of premenopausal women, and 1% of men have an iron deficiency anemia. Approximately 15% of men and women over the age of 60 have iron deficiency, as do 25–40% of nursing home patients. Intestinal blood loss due to tumors or parasites is the primary cause worldwide as compared to nutritive iron deficiency. If the storage iron reserves are exhausted, the transferrin saturation drops below 15% and the soluble transferrin receptor increases intensively. A decrease in the hemoglobin value usually does not occur until 1–2 months later. In patients on oral iron administration, the increased sTfR and the decreased ferritin concentrations normalize within 2–4 weeks (<5 mg/L and >30 µg/L, respectively).

Depending on the pattern of the laboratory test results, it is possible to distinguish between prelatent, latent, and manifest iron deficiencies. In prelatent iron deficiency, the body's iron reserves are reduced. Latent iron deficiency is characterized by a reduced supply of iron for erythropoiesis. This gives way to manifest iron deficiency, which is characterized by typical iron deficiency anemia.

Prelatent iron deficiency, which is equivalent to storage iron deficiency, is characterized by a negative iron balance. The body's reaction is to increase the intestinal absorption of iron. Histochemically, the iron content of bone marrow and of liver tissue decreases. The concentration of the iron transport protein transferrin in the blood increases as a measure of the increased intestinal absorption.

The consumption of storage iron is most easily detected by quantitative determination of the ferritin concentration, which typically falls to less than 20 ng/mL. The ferritin that can be detected in the circulating blood is directly related to the iron stores. Its determination has almost entirely replaced the determination of iron in bone marrow for the assessment of stocks of reserve iron. The determination of the soluble transferrin receptor (sTfR) is becoming increasingly important in the assessment of the erythropoietic activity [117].

With the consumption of reserve iron, or when the iron stores are completely empty, the replenishment of iron for erythropoiesis becomes negative. The total loss of storage iron is indicated by a decrease in the ferritin concentration to less than 12 µg/L. An indication of the inadequate supply of iron for erythropoiesis is a decrease in the transferrin saturation to less than 15%; the sTfR values are above the normal range of >5 mg/L. As a morphologic criterion, the number of sideroblasts in the marrow falls to less than 10%. There are no noticeable changes in the red blood count at this stage of latent iron deficiency.

The laboratory results in the manifest stage are characterized by a fall in the ferritin concentration in the blood to less than 12 µg/L and a fall in the hemoglobin concentration to less than 12 g/dL. A morphologic effect of manifest iron deficiency is that the erythrocytes become increasingly hypochromic and microcytic. The mean cell volume (MCV) decreases to less than 80 fL, the mean cellular hemoglobin (MCH) is less than 28 pg, and the mean cellular hemoglobin concentration (MCHC) may fall to less than 33 g/dL. The erythrocytes in the peripheral blood count are smaller than normal, and pale in the center. These altered erythrocytes are known as anulocytes. The morphologic change in the blood count does not appear immediately, but only after the normochromic erythrocyte population has been replaced by the hypochromic microcytic erythrocytes in the course of the natural process of renewal. Iron deficiency is by no means ruled out by

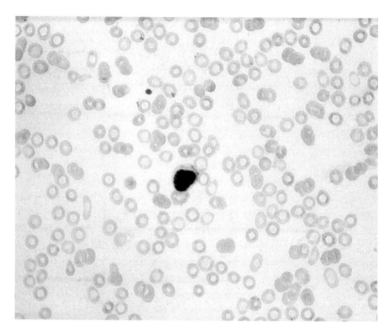

Fig. 25: Anulocytes

normochromic normocytic anemia. Pronounced hypochromia and microcythemia indicate that the iron deficiency has already been in existence for at least several months. This may be microscopically visible as anulocytes (Fig. 25).

A hypochromic microcytic anemia is not necessarily an iron deficiency anemia. However, a morphologically characterized anemia accompanied by a ferritin value of less than 12 µg/L can always be identified as an iron deficiency anemia, and there is then, for the present, no need for further tests (Fig. 26).

It is extremely important in differential diagnosis to distinguish between the common iron deficiency anemias and other hypochromic anemias, since this has considerable implications for therapy. Only iron deficiency anemia responds to iron replacement. For patients suffering from other hypochromic anemias, the unnecessary administration of iron would lead to a risk of iron overload.

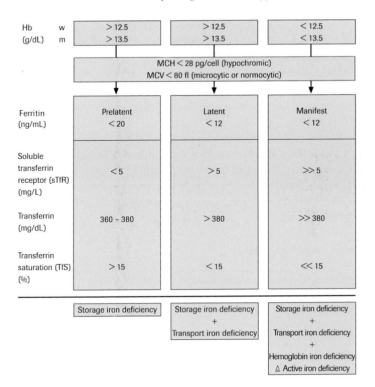

Hb (g/dL)	w m	> 12.5 > 13.5	> 12.5 > 13.5	< 12.5 < 13.5

MCH < 28 pg/cell (hypochromic)
MCV < 80 fl (microcytic or normocytic)

	Prelatent	Latent	Manifest
Ferritin (ng/mL)	< 20	< 12	< 12
Soluble transferrin receptor (sTfR) (mg/L)	< 5	> 5	>> 5
Transferrin (mg/dL)	360 – 380	> 380	>> 380
Transferrin saturation (TfS) (%)	> 15	< 15	<< 15

Storage iron deficiency	Storage iron deficiency + Transport iron deficiency	Storage iron deficiency + Transport iron deficiency + Hemoglobin iron deficiency △ Active iron deficiency

Fig. 26: Laboratory findings in the presence of iron deficiency

Clinical Pictures of Iron Deficiency

Iron deficiency occurs as a sign of increased physiologic iron requirements during growth, as a result of menstruation, in pregnancy, and during breast-feeding. The main cause of pathologic iron deficiency, on the other hand, is loss of blood, usually from the gastrointestinal tract, though also from the urogenital tract in the case of women, and less commonly in both sexes as a result of renal and bladder hemorrhages. Iron deficiency can also be caused by disturbed absorption of iron (malabsorption), in which case it is important to check for any medication that interferes with the absorption of iron. The clinical pictures of latent or manifest iron deficiency following blood loss are relatively easy to be detected by a detailed patient history or by appropriate diagnostic measures. Checks for occult blood in the stools are particularly important in the case of gastrointestinal losses.

Iatrogenic iron deficiency may be caused by excessive laboratory tests or by drugs, such as non-steroidal antirheumatic drugs or antacids. Asymptomatic gastrointestinal losses due to corticosteroids also fall under this heading.

Frequent blood donations (more than 4 times within a year) empty the iron stores. Further donations then lead to a reduced – but constant – ferritin concentration. Males donating 4 or more times per year and females donating 2 or more per year should have at least one ferritin or sTfR determination per year, to allow for the detection and treatment of any prelatent or latent iron deficiency.

Table 16: Causes of iron deficiency

1. Physiologic increase in requirements	3. Malabsorption
• Growth phase • Menstruation • Pregnancy • Breast-feeding	• Sprue • Gastric resections • Chronic atrophic gastritis • Drugs
2. Blood loss	**4. Inadequate supply**

• Gastrointestinal
  – Esophagus
  – Varices
  – Ulcers
  – Tumors
  – Inflammations
  – Malformation (blood vessels)
• Urogenital
  – Hypermenorrhea
  – Birth
  – Tumors of the urinary tract
  – Calculi
• Iatrogenic
  – Laboratory testing (excessive)
  – Drugs
  – Blood donors
	• Unbalanced diet
	• Age
	• New vegetarians

Disturbances of iron absorption are known to occur after gastric resections (often associated with vitamin B_{12} deficiency) and in chronic atrophic gastritis. Malabsorption may also be induced iatrogenically by long-term tetracycline therapy, which is often used for the treatment of acne. Idiopathic sprue generally also leads to iron malabsorption and hence to anemia.

Special consideration must also be given to certain population groups in which iron deficiency is common; these include infants and adolescents, the elderly, competitive athletes, and individuals having an unbalanced diet.

Behavioral disturbances in children can often be traced to latent or manifest iron deficiency. Intellectual and especially cognitive development in childhood is also adversely affected by iron deficiency. The observed symptoms can be eliminated by oral administration of iron. There is some debate as to whether brain development is permanently damaged by iron deficiency in early childhood. Iron deficiency in adolescence, especially in girls, is aggravated by poor eating habits. The supply of iron often corresponds to only 50% of the recommended amount, and this, coupled with puberty, leads to iron deficiency.

Latent iron deficiency is found in more than 50% of all pregnant women. The physiologic course of pregnancy explains why latent iron deficiency appears mainly in the final three months. The ferritin concentration is a reliable parameter for the detection of iron depletion and deficiency in this situation. The daily iron requirement increases to 5–6 mg during the last three months of pregnancy, and this amount cannot be absorbed even from the best possible diet. Oral iron replacement is therefore necessary (Fig. 27).

Iron deficiency in the elderly, particularly those who live alone or in an institution, appears to be caused mainly by diet.

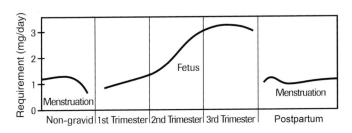

Fig. 27: Iron requirement during pregnancy

Special note should be given to iron deficiency in athletes of both sexes who take part in endurance sports. Iron deficiency in runners is mainly due to gastrointestinal losses after long-distance running. Latent iron deficiency has also been found in long-distance swimmers. In endurance sports, hemolysis apparently is an additional factor.

Extremely unbalanced diets have recently attracted considerable numbers of adherents. Iron deficiency anemia develops here mainly if the diet has an extremely high content of indigestible roughage [25].

Oral Administration of Iron

Oral replacement is always indicated in iron deficiency, which cannot be cured by dietary iron. In spite of various pharmaceutical formulations, the tolerability of oral iron preparations varies a great deal, so that its administration has to be monitored very carefully with regard to patient compliance.

When iron deficiency is present, the absorption of iron is upregulated depending on the iron deficit. A bioavailability of 80–97% is achieved in the stomach and the proximal duodenum, but this requires that iron be supplied in an aqueous solution or released rapidly from the administered preparation. If iron (ferroglycine sulfate) is administered in enteric-coated pellets, about 83% of it is absorbed. If the iron reserves are depleted, this portion can increase to 95% provided that iron is fully released [68]. A slow release of iron reduces absorption and, therefore, the bioavailability by about one-third, to approximately 60%. Iron(III) complexes administered orally are barely bioavailable and are therefore inefficient. The cause of the poor bioavailability lies in the fact that, in the case of iron(III) compounds, complete hydrolysis takes place at pH levels of just 2–4 and polymerization takes place in the small intestine at pH 7–pH 8, forming insoluble and non-absorbable polynuclear iron(III)-hydroxide complexes which, due to their high molecular weight, cannot be absorbed. This reduces the bioavailability to less than 30%.

The bioavailability of oral iron preparations is improved by ingesting it on an empty stomach. The simultaneous consumption of tea, coffee or dairy products in particular reduces the absorption of iron, as demonstrated in absorption studies with ferrous ascorbate solution. In the fasting state, about 10% was absorbed, although only about 1% was absorbed

Table 17: Recommended daily doses for the most common oral iron preparations

Ferrous sulfate	105 mg Fe^{2+}
Ferrous fumarate	308 mg Fe-fumarate $\triangleq$ 100 mg Fe^{2+}
Ferrous gluconate	200 mg Fe-gluconate $\triangleq$ approx. 30 mg Fe^{2+} 625 mg Fe-gluconate/ascorbic acid $\triangleq$ 80 mg Fe^{2+}

after breakfast. The extent of oral absorption is largely unrelated to the pharmaceutical formulation.

The gold standard of therapy is still iron sulfate, which is divided into 1–3 daily doses totalling 100 mg Fe(II). Taken on an empty stomach an iron absorption of 10–20 mg iron per day can be achieved [68]. A significant rise in the hematocrit can be expected within 3 weeks, and a normal red blood count (RBC) can generally be expected after 2 months if no further iron losses occur.

Iron therapy should be continued for a further 3–6 months after reaching a normal level in order to fill the body's iron stores. The ferritin level must be monitored during this period. Ferrous sulfate is suitable for oral administration of iron, as are ferrous sulfate, fumarate, chloride, and lactate.

The most common iron compounds used for oral therapy are listed in Table 17. Fumarate and gluconate, in addition to iron sulfate, are commercially available in presentations ranging from tablets to coated tablets and suspensions. Of the absorption-enhancing substances, only ascorbic acid at a dosage of 200 mg or more has proved to be useful.

Oral iron preparations can cause gastrointestinal side-effects such as heartburn, nausea, flatulence, constipation, and diarrhea. In approximately 25% of the patients, side-effects occur when a daily dosage of more than 100 mg iron is given, regardless of whether they are in the form of three equally divided doses or not. A rise in the side-effect rate to about 50% is observed in test persons when the orally administered iron dosage is doubled. The intensity of the side-effects depends on the dose and the speed at which the iron is released. It is advisable to start therapy with a small dosage and then gradually increase it. Iron preparations with poor bioavailability, therefore, cause relatively few side-effects.

As the intestinal absorption of iron in healthy persons is strictly regulated, it is virtually impossible to bring about symptoms of metal intoxi-

Clinical Aspects

cation by excessive oral administration of iron to adults. Should this nevertheless occur, then hemochromatosis should be looked for. Fatalities in adults following oral administration of iron are generally the result of suicidal intent. The situation is different in children, particularly small children. A dose of just 1 or 2 g of iron can be fatal. Symptoms of iron intoxication can occur within 30 min but may also not develop until several hours have elapsed. They consist of cramp-like abdominal pain, diarrhea, and vomiting of brown or bloody-stained gastric juice. The patients become pale or cyanotic, tired, confused, show incipient hyperventilation as a result of metabolic acidosis and die of cardiovascular failure.

In uncomplicated iron deficiency, hemoglobin or ferritin values increase 2–4 weeks after the start of iron therapy. sTfR reaches a normal level within 2 weeks. The sTfR concentration usually normalizes when ferritin levels >13 (females) or >30 µg/L (males) are reached.

In complicated iron deficiency (infection, inflammation, and malignant tumor), an elevated sTfR concentration decreases as well after successful oral iron therapy. As the ferritin concentration can be normal or increased in the presence of tumor anemia or ACD despite inadequate iron supply for erythropoiesis, the drop in sTfR concentration alone is an indicator that an oral iron therapy is successful.

Parenteral Administration of Iron

The indications for i.v. iron administration are:
- poor iron absorption
- gastrointestinal disorders
- the inability to mobilize adequately large iron stores already present (renal insufficiency)
- intolerance of oral iron administration

Before administering iron parenterally, it is advisable to carry out an approximate calculation of the iron requirement and to administer it taking the iron reserves into account (Tables 18, 19).

Of the preparations available (iron saccharate, iron gluconate, iron dextran, and ferric carboxymaltose), iron saccharate has proved to be the most popular in Europe for parenteral administration. The iron saccharate complex has the advantage that it is not filtered through the

Table 18: Parenteral iron administration. Calculation of total dose to be administered [68]

Total amount of iron (g) = [Hb deficit × blood volume × iron reserve in Hb] + iron deficit in depots	
Example:	**Adult (male)**
Body weight:	70 kg
Blood volume:	0.069 L/kg × body weight
Hb (measured):	90 g/L blood
Hb (deficit):	40 g/L blood
Hb (target):	130 g/L
Iron reserve in Hb:	3.4 mg Fe/g Hb
Iron reserve in depots:	0.5 g (calculated by from ferritin concn.)*
Total iron dose required to increase the Hb value from 9 g/dL to 13 g/dL = $[40 \times 0.069 \times 70 \times 3.4 \times 10^{-3}] + 0.5 = 0.7 + 0.5 = 1.2$ (g)	

*0.5 g iron reserves in the iron depots correspond to a ferritin concentration of approx. 50 ng/mL. As a rule of thumb, 1 ng/mL ferritin equals approx. 10 mg iron in the iron stores.

Table 19: Parenteral iron supplementation of patients under hemodialysis with iron saccharate or iron gluconate

Ferritin Concentration	Iron Saccharate	Iron Gluconate
<100 ng/mL	40 mg Iron/HD*	62.5 mg Iron/HD*
>100 ng/mL	10 mg Iron/HD	10 mg Iron/HD

*Manufacturer's data for contents per bottle; HD hemodialysis.

glomeruli (molecular weight 43,000 D), is therefore not excreted renally and consequently cannot cause a tubulotoxic effect. Furthermore, the substance is characterized by its low potential for triggering an anaphylactic shock. However, in the liver iron is released from the saccharate complex and therefore hepatotoxicity should be watched for as a side-effect. When iron saccharate or iron gluconate is used, the iron doses per hemodialysis listed are acceptable according to the manufacturers' data.

The total dose for remedying a manifest iron deficiency anemia (ferritin <12 ng/mL) is generally between 1.0 and 1.2 g iron administered parenterally.

Clinical Aspects

Megaloblastic and macrocytic anemias as well as iron distribution disturbances, with or without iron deficiency, require more complex therapy.

Side-Effects and Hazards of Parenteral Iron Therapy

During intravenous administration, intolerance reactions (immediately during or after intravenous administration) can occur. Undesired long-term side-effects in various systems of the body have also been described. Accordingly, intravenous iron therapy should only be carried out with strict adherence to the indications.

Immediate reactions include malaise, fever, acute generalized lymph adenopathy, joint pains, urticaria, and occasionally exacerbation of symptoms in patients with rheumatoid arthritis.

These fairly harmless but unpleasant adverse reactions differ from the rare but feared anaphylactic reactions which can be fatal despite immediate therapy. Such reactions with fatal outcome have been reported occasionally particularly for iron dextran. These occurrences necessitate very strict indications for i.v. therapy [31].

There is confirmed evidence that infections, cardiovascular diseases, and carcinogenesis can be influenced by the intravenous administration of iron.

There is a close relationship between the availability of iron and the virulence of bacterial infections. This can be explained by the fact that iron is a precondition for the multiplication of bacteria in the infected body. Excessive iron can therefore increase the risk of infection. It has already been shown in human and animal studies that the intravenous administration of iron during infection causes deterioration of the clinical picture. It has in the meantime been shown that hydroxyl radicals, which are formed during iron therapy, are responsible for the negative effects of iron. In other words, iron deficiency hinders not only bacterial growth but also adequate defense against infection in the affected organism. Particularly in dialysis patients or patients with end-stage renal disease, intravenous iron therapy can negatively influence not only the activity of the phagocytes, but also that of the T- and B-lymphocytes [110].

In patients with malignoma, iron therapy is clearly indicated when iron deficiency exists. However, these patients frequently suffer from ACD in which it is known that functional iron is depressed even though the iron reserves are in the normal or elevated range. Administration of iron when not indicated cannot only have a detrimental effect on various organ systems of the sick person, but may also contribute to increased proliferation of neoplastic cells. Various studies have demonstrated that high transferrin saturation is associated with an elevated risk of carcinoma in general and of cancer of the lungs and colon in particular [93]. In a study comparing the relative cancer risk in blood donors and non-donors, there was a significant increase in the relative risk of non-donors for developing carcinoma [82].

The hypothesis that iron depletion has a protective action against coronary heart disease was advanced as early as 1996 [135] to explain the striking difference between the genders regarding the incidence of coronary heart disease. However, it is still a controversial point of discussion if iron plays a role in the pathogenesis of cardiovascular disease and atherosclerosis.

Ascherio et al. has published a report stating that reduced levels of depot iron do not prevent the risk of coronary disease [8]. The same author reports that an increased dietary intake of hemoglobin iron in men leads to an increased risk of coronary disease even when cholesterol and fat intake are included in the risk assessment [9]. Kiechl et al. observed that serum ferritin values above $50\,\mu g/L$ lead to an increase in atherosclerosis of the carotids in both men and women [81]. Corti et al. [40] reported that the mortality risk and the risk of coronary heart disease increase with low iron levels in individuals over 70 years of age. In dialysis patients it was found that intravenous iron in combination with erythropoietin in dialysis patients increases the cardiovascular risk and, therefore, mortality [21]. Other publications, however, failed to demonstrate significant associations between serum ferritin, transferrin or dietary iron and the developmental stage of an atherosclerosis [54].

The observations supporting the promotion of atherogenesis during intravenous iron therapy led to considerations on the simultaneous use of erythropoietin and desferrioxamine in order to mobilize the iron depots and thus make intravenous administration of iron unnecessary. The difficulty associated with this therapy concept lies in the fact that the mobilization of depot iron cannot be predicted.

In the light of the aspects discussed here, namely the influence of iron on infectious disease, carcinogenesis and the development of atherosclerosis, it seems that stored iron is toxic. Every form of iron therapy therefore requires careful monitoring. The therapeutic goal is the achievement of normal values for hematocrit and hemoglobin.

Clinical Aspects

Disturbances of Iron Distribution and Hypochromic Anemias

Chronic infections, tumors, chronic inflammations, and autoimmune diseases "need" iron and withdraw it from hematopoiesis. "Secondary anemias", "anemias of infection " or "tumor anemias" or anemias of chronic disease (ACD) are the cause of a hypochromic anemia just as often as true iron deficiency. In addition to chronic inflammatory and neoplastic processes, they are observed primarily in patients with extensive tissue trauma. They are observed in the presence of chronic inflammatory and neoplastic processes as well as extensive tissue injuries.

While in patients with primary and secondary hemochromatoses the plasma ferritin concentration correlates with the body's total iron stores, there are other conditions in which this correlation does not apply. Raised plasma ferritin concentrations are also found in patients with toxin-induced damage to the liver resulting from ferritin release by necrotic liver cells, in patients with latent and manifest inflammations or infections, and in patients with rheumatoid arthritis. In addition, raised plasma ferritin concentrations are observed in patients suffering from physical and psychologic stress, e.g. following serious trauma. In critically ill patients, plasma ferritin concentrations increase with increasing deterioration of the patient's clinical status, probably as a result of increased release from the macrophage system [23] (Table 20, Fig. 28).

Table 20: Causes of iron displacement in patients with secondary anemias

Infections	• Chronic bronchitis • Chronic urinary tract infection • Chronic varicose complex or gangrene • Osteomyelitides • Tuberculosis
Tumors	• Carcinomas • Sarcoma • Lymphoma • Leukemia • Plasmocytoma
Autoimmune diseases	• Collagenoses • Rheumatoid diseases
Toxic effects	• Multiple drug and environmentally related effects

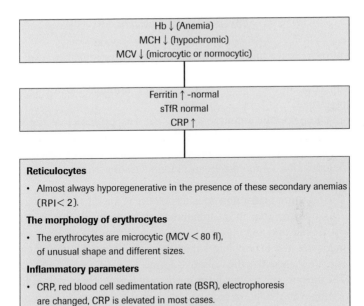

Hb ↓ (Anemia)
MCH ↓ (hypochromic)
MCV ↓ (microcytic or normocytic)

Ferritin ↑ -normal
sTfR normal
CRP ↑

Reticulocytes

- Almost always hyporegenerative in the presence of these secondary anemias (RPI< 2).

The morphology of erythrocytes

- The erythrocytes are microcytic (MCV < 80 fl),
  of unusual shape and different sizes.

Inflammatory parameters

- CRP, red blood cell sedimentation rate (BSR), electrophoresis
  are changed, CRP is elevated in most cases.

Causes of secondary anemia in the presence of iron redistribution

are infections, liver diseases or tumors;
Iron moves into the reticular tissue instead to hematopoiesis

Fig. 28: Further laboratory findings in patients with secondary hypochromic anemias

The plasma ferritin concentration is not indicative of the body's total iron stores shortly after oral or parenteral iron therapy, or in patients with malignant tumors. As a basic rule, it can be assumed that a raised red blood cell sedimentation rate and/or pathologic values for C-reactive protein (CRP) are likely to be accompanied by raised plasma ferritin concentrations.

The characteristics of these anemias are a low serum iron concentration combined with a low transferrin saturation and a sTfR in the normal range; ferritin is available in sufficient or elevated quantities and the morphology of the anemia is normocytic or microcytic.

Iron and Cellular Immunity

The purpose of the immune system is to protect the organism from microorganisms, foreign substances, harmful substances, toxins, and malignant cells. A non-specific and a specific immune defense can be distinguished.

The non-specific immune system consists primarily of the acid mantle of the skin, intact epidermis, intact complement system, antimicrobial enzyme systems, and non-specific mediators such as interferons and interleukins. Granulocytes and monocytes/macrophages act at the cellular level.

The most important non-specific defense is the inflammatory reaction. As the first step in an inflammatory reaction, mediators (IL-1, IFN-γ) are released and increase the permeability of the capillary walls. Granulocytes and macrophages then enter the source of inflammation in order to phagocytize the causative agent.

The purpose of the specific immune system is to expand the antigen by cloning when inflammation occurs to enable a memory reaction in the future. T-lymphocytes formed in the thymus and B-lymphocytes formed in the bone marrow are specialized for this in particular. The maturation of T-lymphocytes takes place upon contact with dendritic cells and macrophages. This maturation process in the IL-12/IFN-γ cytokine environment results in CD4+-THO cells and, finally, TH1 cells. The TH1 cells play a key role in the pathogenesis of disturbances of iron utilization in the presence of tumor anemias and anemias of infection, and chronic inflammation (Fig. 29).

Dendritic cells (DC) are the most important cells of non-specific immunity in the body. T-cells are able to stimulate immature DC to a limited extent; they are finally induced to mature into dendritic cells when affected by the inflammatory-acting cytokines TNF-c, IL-1, IL-6, LPS (lipopolysaccharide), bacteria, and viruses.

Only terminally mature dendritic cells (DC) that were stimulated by CD40/CD40 ligands are able to produce large amounts of IL-12. This cytokine, in turn, induces the differentiation of CD4+-THO cells in the direction of TH1 with the release of interferon. Interferon-γ stimulates the antimicrobial and proinflammatory activity of macrophages and helps further the activation of cytotoxic T-cells (cytotoxic T-lymphocytes, CTL).

Clinical Aspects

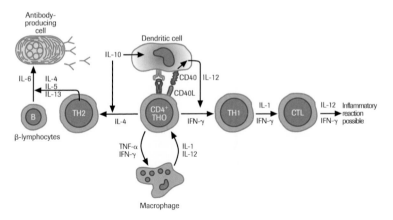

Fig. 29: Cell–cell interaction of cytokines in the differentiation of TH0 into TH1 and TH2 cells. According to [30, 74, 134]

Interleukins: IL-4, IL-5, IL-6, IL-10, IL-12, IL-13
IFN-γ: Interferon γ
CTL: Cytotoxic T-lymphocytes
TH0, TH1, TH2: Subpopulations of T-lymphocytes
CD40, CD40L: Cluster of differentiation (CD) 40 and 40L (according to the WHO-IUIS-Standardization Committee of Leukocyte Differentiation Antigens)
B: B-Lymphocyte
TNF-α: Tumor necrosis factor alpha

TH1 cells secrete interleukin-2, interferon-γ, TNF-α, and GM-CSF and result, via macrophage activation, in pronounced inflammatory processes that enable the destruction of intracellular causative agents. The activation of macrophages results in the secretion of increased amounts of TNF-α. This reduces the production of antibodies and cell-destroying enzymes. Both of these induce an increase in TNF-α synthesis.

In the non-terminal differentiation of CD, e.g., when the T-cells do not express the CD40 ligands, or in the presence of IL-10, the differentiation of T-cells leans toward TH2, with the secretion of IL-4 and IL-5. Together with IL-13 and IL-6, these cytokines induce the maturation of B-cells in antibody-producing plasma cells, and the inflammatory cytotoxic T-cell response does not take place.

As illustrated in Fig. 30, the subpopulation of CD4+-T helper cells (TH1) releases pro-inflammatory cytokines, which have a direct

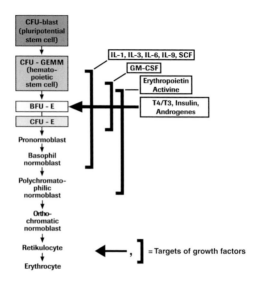

Fig. 30. Differentiation of the hematopoietic system and regulation of erythropoiesis by growth factors

CFU, colony-forming unit; BFU, burst-forming unit; GEMM, granulocytic erythrocytotic, macrophagocytic, megaloblastic; IL, Interleukin; SCF, stem cell factor; GM-CSF, granulocyte-macrophage colony-stimulating factor.

effect on iron metabolism, while the TH2 population is mainly responsible for the antibody response and does not directly affect iron metabolism.

The cytokines produced by TH1 subsets, such as interleukin-1 (IL1) and tumor necrosis factor alpha (TNF-α), induce ferritin synthesis in cells of the non-specific immune system such as macrophages and hepatocytes, while interferon gamma (IFN-γ) withholds iron from the macrophages [149].

Increased release of cytokines such as IFN-γ and TNF-α, mediated by nitrogen oxide (NO), leads to an increased iron uptake in macrophages by an increased transferrin receptor expression. The increased iron uptake induces increased intracellular ferritin synthesis.

Iron intervenes in cellular immunity at many levels [151]. On the one hand, it affects the proliferation and differentiation of various lym-

phocyte subsets. On the other, it affects the immunopotential of macrophages [26, 43] by blocking the IFN-γ-transmitted immune response
in macrophages. Iron-overloaded macrophages react more poorly to
IFN-γ, produce more TNF-α, and form more NO.

The ceruloplasmin/haptoglobin system lowers NO and directly affects the proliferation of the precursor cells of erythropoiesis. Additionally, the resistance to viruses and other intracellular pathogens is
weakened. The withdrawal of metabolically active iron and its deposit as
storage iron strengthen the organism's immune response to IFN-stimu-
lation [22, 103].

The regulatory antagonist of this stimulation mechanism lies in the
decrease of the TH1-mediated immune reaction by IL-4 and IL-13. This
is accomplished when these interleukins raise the intracellular concentration of iron by stimulating transferrin receptor expression. This is
one of the basic mechanisms of the anti-inflammatory and macrophage-
inhibiting effect [103].

Activation of the Immunological and Inflammatory Systems

Anemias of chronical disease (ACD) are the result of a multifactorial
process in which activation of the immune and inflammatory systems
and the iron metabolism in monocytes/macrophages play an important
role (Fig. 31).

The anti-inflammatory and anti-neoplastic defense mechanisms
draw iron from microorganisms and neoplastic cells and store it in the
reticuloendothelial system. This is complicated by the development of a
normo-chromic or hypochromic anemia. These types of anemia are
caused by tumors, malignant growths, and chronic inflammations. Due
to various cytokines, erythropoiesis is compromised primarily at the
CFU-E level in this process.

Erythropoietin (EPO) is the most important and specific erythropoiesis-stimulating factor. It acts on early progenitor cells up to the
maturation levels after the erythroblast stage. Without EPO, erythroid
differentiation does not progress past the level of burst-forming units
(BFU-E).

The progenitor cells of the red line proliferate and differentiate
only under optimal local conditions. The blood formation islands in

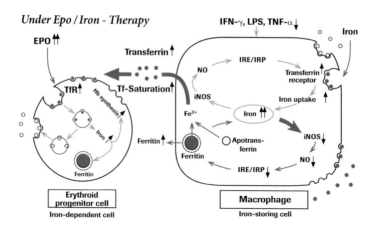

Fig. 31: Iron supply of an iron-dependent cell in a patient on EPO/iron therapy. Modified according to [150]

IFN-γ, interferon γ; iNOS, inducible nitric oxide synthase; IRE, iron-responsive element; IRE/IRP high-affinity binding of iron-regulatory protein (IRP) to IREs; LPS, lipopolysaccharide; TNF-α, tumor necrosis factor-α; ↑ and ↓ indicate increase or decrease of cellular responses, respectively.

∪ transferrin receptor, • iron-carrying transferrin, ○ apotransferrin, ○ ferritin

bone marrow consist of a centrally located macrophage surrounded by small cells of the erythroid and myeloid line. The surrounding cells also comprise endothelial cells, fat cells, reticuloepithelial cells, and fibroblasts [151]. High concentrations of intracellular iron dramatically reduce the effect of IFN-γ on human monocytic cells. Iron regulates the cytokine effects in this process. Macrophages with high concentrations of intracellular iron lose the ability to phagocyte. After stimulation with IFN- and lipopolysaccharides (LPS), cultivated macrophages produce increasing quantities of nitrogen oxide (NO), which is then converted to reactive nitrogen intermediates (RNI) such as nitrite and nitrate (Fig. 31).

An undesired effect in particular is the fact that availability of iron for hemoglobin synthesis is reduced. Iron replacement as part of erythropoietin therapy stimulates erythropoiesis and iron uptake by the bone marrow cells on the one hand, and, on the other, withdraws iron from the macrophages and reduces the cytotoxic effects [153].

Table 21: Biochemical background of EPO/iron combination therapy

	Erythroid cells	**Reticuloendothelial system (e.g., macrophages)**
EPO ↑ = EPO treatment	stimulates proliferation of bone marrow erythroid cells and upregulates TfR expression	upregulates transferrin receptor expression
"Free iron" ↑ = i.v. iron treatment	stimulates Hb synthesis	inhibits NOS and NO production, upregulates ferritin expression, and inhibits IFN-γ and TNF-α production

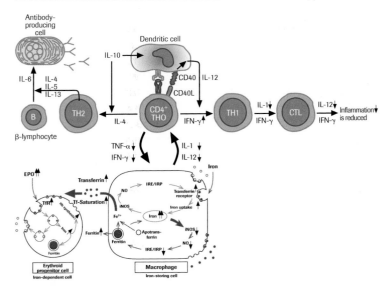

Fig. 32: Differentiation of T-cells into TH1- and TH2-cells' role of cytokines in the cell–cell interaction

IFN-γ, interferon-γ; TNF-α, tumor necrosis factor-α; NO, nitric oxide; iNOS, inducible nitric oxide synthase; IL, interleukin; IRE, iron-responsive element; IRP, iron-regulatory protein; Tf, transferrin; TfR, transferrin receptor

The combination of iron and erythropoietin therapy is favorable, since in addition to improving the anemia, the previously described inhibiting effect of iron on cytokine action and macrophage-induced cytotoxicity has a positive influence.

With erythropoietin administration, the transferrin receptor on erythroid precursor cells is upregulated. A sequential administration of erythropoietin and iron (at intervals of 48 hours) is recommended [149].

It is possible that a combination of EPO/i.v. iron leads to a reduction of iron deposits in the macrophages and downregulates the cytokine interaction and the inflammatory reaction, primarily of IL-1, IL-12, and IFN-γ, while the inflammatory activity is simultaneously inhibited (Fig. 32). This would explain the inflammation-inhibiting effect of combined EPO therapy and i.v. iron administration. When one considers that the therapy has no side-effects and that it leads not only to correction of anemia in patients with tumors and infections and in patients with chronic inflammation (e.g., rheumatoid arthritis), but also to a correction in the inflammatory activity, it becomes clear that an important milestone in the therapy of these diseases has been reached.

Therapy with Erythropoietin and i.v. Iron Administration

The first ESAs (erythropoiesis-stimulating agents) were recombinant human erythropoietin (epoetin alpha and beta) which could be administered either intravenously (i.v.) or subcutaneously (s.c.), and were generally given two or three times a week. The frequency of administration was dictated partly by the short biologic half-life of these products – about 6–8 hours following a single i.v. injection [95].

In addition to rhu-EPO (recombinant human erythropoietin), recombinant DNA technology has made it possible to synthesize an analog to rhu-EPO, the Novel Erythropoiesis-Stimulating Protein (NESP), darbopoietin alpha [47, 94]. This molecule was created by the addition of two extra N-linked carbohydrate chains, increasing the total number of sialic acid residues and conferring additional metabolic stability on the molecule. Thus, the elimination half-life of i.v. darbopoietin alpha in humans was three times longer than that of standard epoetin, which makes longer administration intervals possible [47]. 200 IU rhu-EPO is roughly equivalent to 1 μg NESP. Antibodies to NESP have yet to be detected in the serum of treated patients [58].

Even more recently, a third generation erythropoietic molecule, Continuous Erythropoietin Receptor Activator (C.E.R.A.), was created

Table 22: Mean half-lives of erythropoiesis-stimulating agents. Continuous Erythropioietion Receptor Activator (C.E.R.A.), darbopoietin alpha, epoietin beta, and epoietin alpha [95]

Agent	Administration route	Mean (± SEM) half-life (h)
Epoietin α	Intravenous	6.8 ± 0.6
	Subcutanous	19.4 ± 2.5
Epoietin β	Intravenous	8.8 ± 0.5
	Subcutanous	24.2 ± 2.6
Darbopoietin α	Intravenous	25.3 ± 2.2
	Subcutanous	48.8 ± 5.2
C.E.R.A.	Intravenous	134 ± 19
	Subcutanous	139 ± 20

by integrating a large polymer chain into the molecule, thus increasing the molecular weight to twice of that of epoietin at approximately 60 kD. This methoxy-polyethylene glycol polymer chain is integrated via amide bonds between the N-terminal amino group or the ε-amino group of lysine (predominantly lysine-52 or lysine-45), using a single succinimidyl butanoic acid linker [95].

Evidence is accumulating that C.E.R.A. has very different receptor-binding characteristics and pharmacokinetic properties from either epoietin or darbopoietin alpha. It has a much lower affinity for the erythropoietin receptor compared with the natural ligand, leading to reduced specific activity in vitro. Because the elimination of half-life is so prolonged, however, C.E.R.A. has increased erythropoietic activity in vivo.

The clinical picture of renal anemia is a "classic" example for replacement therapy with rhu-EPO. Nor is it surprising that over 95% of dialysis patients are successfully treated with rhu-EPO [136].

Under physiologic conditions, the neogenesis of erythropoietin takes place in the peritubular fibroblasts of the kidney. Under hypoxic conditions, synthesis of the hormone – mediated by a cellular oxygen sensor – increases (rise in the expression of the EPO gene). In patients with chronic renal insufficiency, these kidney cells lose their ability to adequately increase EPO formation.

There are a number of forms of anemia that are not due primarily to a deficit of EPO, but which can be corrected using rhEPO therapy. Almost all chronic inflammatory or malignant diseases are associated with an anemia. Many factors are significant with these anemias. First and

Clinical Aspects

Table 23: Summary of EPO features

Formation site	• Specialized kidney cells • Regenerating human liver cells
Regulation by	• Hormones such as renin, angiotensin II or epinephrine • Cytokines such as IL-1, IL-6 or TNF • Oxygen supply at the site of EPO production
Biologic function	• Growth factor • Promotion of proliferation and differentiation of erythrocyte precursor cells
EPO in disease	• In patients with certain forms of anemia, especially aplastic anemia, the regulation of EPO formation in the kidneys appears to be intact. This leads to extremely high EPO concentrations in the serum of the individuals affected (up to 4 U/mL). Other forms of anemia, especially renal anemia, are characterized by serum EPO concentrations that are lower than expected for the severity of the anemia. The regulation of EPO formation is apparently disturbed in these individuals. • Forms of anemia that may or may not be based on a deficit of erythropoietin. This question can be clarified by determining the erythropoietin concentration in serum and by relating the results to the hemoglobin concentration (or the hematocrit). • Elevated values of erythropoietin accompanied by a normal or even raised hemoglobin concentration (and/or hematocrit values) were found in a number of diseases such as kidney and liver tumors or in patients with secondary forms of polycythemia. Polycythemia vera is characterized by an abnormally high number of red blood cells accompanied by a reduced serum titer of erythropoietin.

foremost, the formation of red blood cells in the bone marrow is disturbed. Circulating cytokines released as part of the inflammatory process are responsible for causing the inhibition of erythropoiesis (TNF-α, IL-1, and IL-6).

In patients with tumor anemias, anemias of infection, or anemias of chronic inflammatory diseases, the direct inhibition of erythropoiesis and the reduced formation of erythropoietin caused by the circulating cytokines, or the reduced release of iron from the reticuloendothelial system means that higher EPO doses are required to correct the anemia as compared to renal anemia. In many patients with carcinomas, infections or chronic intestinal disease or rheumatoid arthritis, however, the hematocrit can be increased, the need for transfusions can be reduced, and quality of life can be improved.

Anemias of Infection and Malignancy

The anemia of infections and malignancies, and anemia of chronic disease (ACD) are observed with greater frequency in internal medical practices than iron deficiency anemia. These anemias are caused by disturbances of iron distribution with insufficient recycling of iron from the storage iron compartment into the functional compartment. The erythropoietic precursor cells are supplied with inadequate amounts of iron even though the RES is filled with iron.

The hypoproliferation of erythropoiesis is induced by inflammatory cytokines (IL-1, IL-6, and TNF-α). The erythropoiesis is adjusted for the reduced iron supply, so that normal hemoglobinization of the red blood cells takes place. This results in a normocytic, normochromic anemia with low erythrocyte count.

The clinical findings in patients with anemias of inflammation and malignancy are presented in Table 24. If these patients experience bleed-

Table 24: Clinical findings in patients with anemia of infection, inflammation and malignancy, and clinical interpretation

Clinical findings		Clinical interpretation
Hemoglobin	9–12 g/dL	Normochromic, normocytic anemia. If
MCH	>28 pg	accompanied by inadequate iron supply
Erythrocytes	3–4 mill./L	for erythropoiesis, hypochromic and
MCV	>80 fL	microcyticerythrocytes are formed.
Reticulocyte Production Index	<2	Hypoproliferative erythropoiesis caused by a reduced erythropoietin effect.
Iron	40 µg/dL	Disturbance of iron distribution due to
Ferritin	100 µg/L	increasing storage in the macrophages of
Transferrin	<200 mg/dL	the reticuloendothelial system.
Transferrin saturation	<15%	
sTfR normal		

MCH: mean cell hemoglobin; MCV: mean cell volume; sTfR: soluble transferrin receptor

Clinical Aspects

ing, however, a combination of iron deficiency and anemia of inflammation or malignancy may occur. Diagnosis of an active iron deficiency is difficult in such cases and cannot be clarified based on the laboratory parameters ferritin and transferrin saturation. However, soluble transferrin receptor (sTfR) may contribute to diagnosis in these cases.

Biologic Activity of Tumor Necrosis Factor

Monocytes and macrophages are the main source of Tumor Necrosis factor (TNF). TNF induces a series of proinflammatory changes in endothelial cells as well as the production of additional proinflammatory cytokines, the expression of adhesion molecules, the release of procoagulatory substance, and the induction of iNOS (inducible nitric oxide synthase) [150].

The therapeutic success of blocking antibodies and receptor fusion proteins [125] underscores the importance of searching for further therapeutic agents with the goal of effectively inhibiting TNF effects:

- Substances that inhibit the formation of TNF, such as phosphodiesterase inhibitors, prostaglandins, adenosine, corticosteroids, and interleukin-10.
- Substances that prevent the processing of the TNF-pro protein by inhibiting the specific metalloproteinase.
- Substances that weaken the effect of the active TNF such as anti-TNF antibodies and TNF receptor Fc fusion proteins.

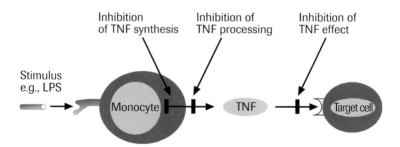

Fig. 33: The biologic activities of TNF [92]

Hemoglobin in Therapies with Cytostatic Drugs

Randomized studies in patients with multiple myeloma (MM), non-Hodgkin's lymphoma (NHL) or chronic lymphatic leukemia (CLL) have made it clear that administration of EPO can raise hemoglobin and reduce a patient's need for transfusions [34, 91].

The hemoglobin value (Hb) is apparently an important factor in the quality of life in patients on virtually any cytostatic therapy. A large multicentric, randomized study conducted by Littlewood et al. [91] investigated the influence of EPO on the need for transfusions and the quality of life of patients with solid tumors and hematologic system diseases under chemotherapy that does not include cis-platinum. The study included patients with solid tumors or hematologic neoplasias in which anemia (Hb < 10.5 g/dL) was diagnosed or in which the Hb value fell by more than 1.5 g/dL in the first four weeks of chemotherapy. The patients were treated with rhEPO (3 × 150 IU/kg/week) for 28 weeks in parallel with chemotherapy. Despite the chemotherapy, treatment with erythropoietin led to an increase in the hemoglobin value by 2 g/dL, in patients with solid tumors as well as patients with hematologic neoplasias.

Anemias in the presence of malignant tumors are therefore the result of a multifactorial process in which the immune system and the inflammatory process play a dominant role [93].

Known causes of anemias in patients with neoplasias are tumor-induced bleeding, hemolysis or infiltration of the bone marrow by tumor cells. The majority of anemias that occur in conjunction with malignant neoplasias are caused either directly or indirectly by the tumor itself, however. Anemia is the result of an imbalance between the rate of production of erythrocytes in the bone marrow and their residence time in the blood. The tumor impairs the proliferation and life span of red blood cells. It is known that the life span of erythrocytes is shortened from 120 days to 60–90 days in patients with malignancies. The activation of the immune system in tumor-induced anemia apparently leads to a suppression of erythropoiesis, for which cytokines are responsible (TNF-α, IL-1, and IFN-γ).

The activation of erythropoiesis is regulated by erythropoietin produced in the proximal tubuli of the kidney. In patients with tumor-induced anemias, exogenously supplied recombinant erythropoietin stimulates the proliferation and differentiation of the red

Clinical Aspects

blood cells precursors. Erythropoietin and IFN-γ can be considered opponents in terms of their effect on erythropoiesis. IFN-γ inhibits the expression of the erythropoietin receptor. It is therefore understandable that recombinant erythropoietin counteracts the tumor-induced anemia.

The hemoglobin level above all is a prognostic factor. This was determined more than 10 years ago in patients with small-cell lung carcinoma. The participation of the bone marrow and the residual hematopoiesis – not the type of tumor – apparently are decisive factors in the success of therapy, as are the type, duration, and intensity of chemotherapy. Chemotherapy schemes that contain platinol compounds exhibit a better reaction to erythropoietin doses. Interestingly enough, a low initial erythropoietin value, as one often finds primarily in patients with lymphoma and myeloma, is a good prognostic factor for a patient's response to therapy. An initial erythropoietin level of less than 250 IU/L is considered particularly favorable.

The prognosis of therapeutic success with solid tumors is more difficult, although a rise in the sTfR within two weeks after onset of therapy is considered a favorable prediction for therapeutic success. Ludwig et al. [93] report therapeutic successes in which an increase in hemoglobin concentration by more than 0.5 g/dL and a drop in the erythropoietin level to less than 100 IU/L was observed after 2 weeks.

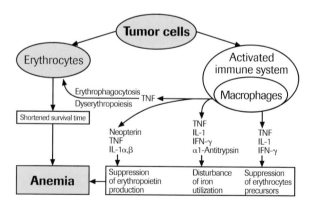

Fig. 34: Pathophysiologic mechanisms in tumor-induced anemia. Modified according to [108] TNF: tumor necrosis factor; IFN: interferon; IL: interleukin.

A drop in serum ferritin is also interpreted as a favorable sign for the therapy.

In the mean time, patients on radiotherapy have also been treated with erythropoietin. It was observed that the hemoglobin value increased among the patients with EPO, but it did not in the untreated control group.

Hypoxic regions exhibit increased resistance to radiation therapy. Apparently there is a correlation between the Hb value and the median oxygen partial pressure in the tumors. Since the hemoglobin concentration is the most important oxygen-supply-determining parameter, an increase in the Hb value with EPO to over 12 g/dL in oncologic patients appears reasonable, even if non-oncologic patients typically are still capable of tolerating lower Hb values.

Erythropoietin and Iron Replacement in Tumor Anemias

Patients with malignant diseases often develop an anemia that is caused by the malignant process itself or the therapy. Various factors such as the type of tumor and the duration of illness, as well as the type and intensity of chemotherapy and/or radiotherapy influence the anemia rate.

Nearly 50–60% of patients who undergo aggressive chemotherapy to treat a malignant lymphoma, bronchial carcinoma, gynecologic tumors or a carcinoma of the urogenital tract require blood transfusions. Blood transfusions are associated with numerous side-effects and risks, however (such as allergic reactions or infections such as hepatitis, HIV, bacterial contamination of the blood product or a blood group incompatibility). An unavoidable side-effect of blood transfusions is chronic immune suppression. This is fatal in tumor patients in particular, as it can encourage tumor progression. Other side-effects include iron and volume overload.

These disadvantages can be prevented by administering recombinant human erythropoietin. EPO increases the Hb value in the physiologic pathway and leads to improved quality of life in patients. EPO administration is therefore better tolerated and has a favorable influence on the results of cancer treatment. Tumor hypoxia and anemia are negative prognostic indicators in terms of the results of treatment of solid and hematologic tumors.

Clinical Aspects

The treatment of anemia while simultaneously reducing transfusions is already being used, in addition to chemotherapy treatment, very successfully in patients

- with solid tumors
- with malignant lymphomas (e.g., chronic lymphatic leukemia [CLL], Hodgkin's lymphoma [HL], non-Hodgkin's lymphoma [NHL])
- with multiple myeloma (MM)
- who have an increased transfusion risk due to their general condition (e.g., cardiovascular status and anemia)
- on chemotherapy with platinum derivatives and chemotherapy drugs that do not contain platinum.

As a result of a patient's response to therapy with erythropoietin, the need for erythrocyte concentrate transfusions drops substantially. In a clinical study conducted by Leon et al. [87] to analyze the erythrocyte requirement under chemotherapy, only 16% of patients treated with erythropoietin required a transfusion. The same observation was described by Qvist et al. [118].

Clinical experience shows that the following response rates are obtained under a dosage of erythropoietin of 150 IU/kg body weight (approx. 10,000 IU), 3 times a week:

Table 25: Percentage of malignancy patients with endogenous EPO deficiency and response rates to rhu-EPO therapy

Clinical picture	Endogenous erythropoietin deficiency [%]	Response rates to recombinant erythropoietin [%]
NHL	38	50–61
CLL	53	approx. 50
CMS	59	Variable
MM	80	50–80
MDS	–	8–28
Solid tumors	86	40–62
After chemotherapy	50–80	52–82

NHL: Non-Hodgkin's lymphoma
CLL: Chronic lympathic lymphoma
CMS: Chronic myeloproliferative syndrome
MM: Multiple myeloma
MDS: Myelodysplastic syndrome

Clinical Aspects

According to this information, more than half of the patients with NHL, CLL or MM respond very well to erythropoietin treatment. Good to very good response rates are typically found in patients with solid tumors and with chemotherapy-induced anemias as well.

The response rates in patients with myelodysplastic syndrome (MDS), in contrast, is low, i.e., less than 10%. This is likely due to the fact that a disturbance of iron utilization exists here. Investigations conducted by Mantovani [99] indicate that erythropoietin does not affect the immunologic parameters IL-1, IL-6, or TNF-α in these tumor patients.

The following indications for treatment with erythropoietin in patients with malignancies are clinically promising (Table 26):

Table 26: Indications for EPO treatment of malignancies

- Prevention of iatrogenic hemosiderosis and transfusion reactions
- Multiple myeloma (MM) when serum erythropoietin is below 100 IU/L
- Non-Hodgkin's lymphoma (NHL), Hodgkin's disease with bone marrow infiltration, and therapy with monoclonal antibodies
- Myelodysplastic syndrome (MDS) when serum erythropoietin is below 100 IU/L
- Chronic Myeloproliferative syndrome (CMS), depending on the extent of bone marrow insufficiency

The most important predictive parameter for response to EPO therapy is functional iron deficiency (ferritin > 20 µg/L, sTfR > 5 mg/L). Functional iron deficiency is one of the most important factors that influence the response to EPO. Elimination of the functional iron deficiency is best accomplished by parenteral iron substitution with a ferrous saccharate complex.

Further important predictors at the onset of therapy are the endogenous EPO serum level and the thrombocyte count. Low serum erythropoietin values at the onset of therapy (<250 IU/L) and normal thrombocyte counts (>100 × 109/L) are therefore independent prognostic factors that indicate a response.

Beginning in week 2–4, relative changes in reticulocytes, the Hb value, and the transferrin receptors in the serum represent good starting points. The prediction as to whether the patient will respond to EPO or not makes it possible to achieve maximum effectiveness and, therefore, to minimize costs.

The therapy of anemias of infections, tumors, and chronic inflammation is characterized by inadequate erythropoietin secretion and can be effectively corrected by the use of rhu-EPO or NESP when the functional iron deficiency was eliminated concomitantly by iron doses.

The recommended erythropoietin dose is approximately 150 IU rhu-EPO/kg body weight three times a week. This corresponds to about 450 IU rhu-EPO/kg body weight once a week. For 70 kg/body weight, this works out to about 31,000 IU rhu-EPO or 15 µg NESP.

Recent investigations have shown that the administration of 150 U/kg body weight of erythropoietin i.v. three times a week can be replaced with a dose of approximately 30,000 IU subcutaneously once a week beginning with chemotherapy.

Hemoglobin increases under this therapeutic regimen, and the transfusion requirement drops dramatically. In a study conducted by Cheung [37], the clinical effect and similar pharmacodynamics were observed with equally good clinical results. The same observations were reported in a study by Gabrilove [55], in which patients reported a distinct improvement in quality of life, which was significantly related to the rise in hemoglobin concentration.

In the present studies, the one-time high-dosage administration of erythropoietin shows the same results as the dose three times a week, but it clearly has the advantage that patient care is more pleasant. It is

Table 27: Combined doses of EPO/i.v. iron in the treatment of tumor anemias

EPO (IU/week)	Approx. 30,000
i.v. iron (mg/week)	<20
Target Hb (g/dL)	12
Target ferritin (µg/L)	100–300
Target sTfR (mg/L)	<5
Target TfS (%)	>15
Target CRP (mg/L)	<5

ACD: Anemia of chronic disease
TfS: Transferrin saturation
sTfR: Soluble transferrin receptor
Hb: Hemoglobin
CRP: C-reactive protein

Clinical Aspects

Table 28: Diagnostic parameters and targets for iron replacement in patients with tumor anemia under EPO therapy

Diagnostic parameter	Expected values	Frequency of determination
Hemoglobin	12 g/dL	
Hematocrit	30–36%	Initially and then quarterly
Reticulocytes	10–15‰	
Folate	20 ng/mL	
Vitamin B$_{12}$	>2 ng/mL	Semi-annually
Ferritin	100–300 ng/mL	
Soluble transferrin receptor	>5 mg/L	
Transferrin saturation	20–30%	At the beginning and then quarterly
Hypochromic erythrocytes	<10%	
CRP	<5 mg/L	

likely that the intervals of the once-per-week administration of NESP can be extended.

In order to best care for patients who receive rhu-EPO in combination with i.v. Fe(III) injections, the essential diagnostic parameters of iron metabolism should be determined at regular intervals during treatment (Table 28).

All hematologic parameters and iron parameters should be determined at the onset of therapy with rhu-EPO and with i.v. iron. These parameters should be tested quarterly.

In 2007 an update of the EORTC (European Organisation for Research and Treatment of Cancer) guidelines for the use of erythropoietic proteins in anemic patients with cancer was published [1]. The following recommendations were offered for anemia management in adult cancer patients with solid tumors or hematologic malignancies:

- Causes of anemia other than cancer or its treatment should be evaluated. Iron deficiency, nutritional defects, bleeding, or hemolysis should be corrected prior to erythropoietic protein therapy. Functional iron deficiency should be addressed with intraveneous iron.
- In cancer patients receiving chemotherapy and/or radiotherapy, treatment with erythropoietic proteins should be initiated at Hb level of 9–11 g/dL based on anemia-related symptoms.
- In patients with cancer-related anemia not undergoing chemotherapy and/or radiotherapy, treatment with erythropoietic proteins

should be initiated at Hb level of 9–11 g/dL based on anemia-related symptoms.

- Patients whose Hb level is below 9 g/dL should be evaluated for need of transfusions, in addition to erythropoietc proteins.
- Erythropoietic proteins may be considered in asymptomatic, anemic patients with a Hb level of <11.9 mg/dL to prevent a further decline in Hb, according to individual factors (e.g., type/intesity of chemotherapy, baseline Hb) and the duration and type of further planned treatment.
- The prophylactic use of erythropoietic proteins to prevent anemia in patients undergoing chemotherapy and/or radiotherapy is not recommended.
- There is no evidence to increased response to erythropoietic proteins with the addition of oral iron supplementation. There is evidence of improved response to erythropoietic proteins with i.v. iron supplementation.
- Based on clinical evidence, elderly patients experience the same benefits from treatment with erythropoietic proteins as younger patients.
- The target Hb concentration should be 12–13 g/dL.
- The administration of erythropoietic proteins according to Fig. 35 is recommended. Dose-escalation as a general approach in patients not responding within 4–8 weeks is not recommended.
- Treatment should be continued until the 12–13 g/dL level of Hb is reached and patients show symptomatic improvement. For patients reaching the target Hb, individualized treatment with increased intervals of dosing and/or titration of the lowest effective maintenance dose should be made repeatedly.
- The use of higher than licensed initial doses of epoietin alpha, epoietin beta, or darbopoietin alpha is not recommended.
- There are no predictive factors of response to erythropoietic proteins that can be routinely used in clinical practice if functional iron deficiency or vitamin deficiency is ruled out. A low serum EPO level (in particular in hematologic malignancies) is the only verified predictive factor of some importance. Values must be interpreted relative to the degree of anemia present. Further studies are needed to define the value of hepcidin and CRP.

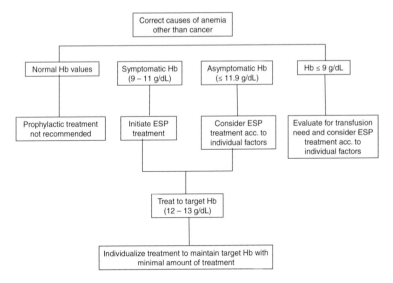

Fig. 35: Proposed dosing algorithm for erythropoietic proteins in patients with cancer with anemia due to cancer or its treatment

ESP, erythropoiesis-stimulating protein.

Anemias of Chronic Inflammatory Processes

The cellular immune system (granulocytes, monocytes/macrophages, natural killer cells, T- and B-lymphocytes) is involved in all inflammatory processes and especially in chronic inflammations such as infections, malignant growth, and skeletal diseases such as rhematoid arthritis, collagenoses, and autoimmune diseases.

After the discovery of the proinflammatory proteins interleukin-1 (IL-1) and tumor necrosis factor alpha (TNF-α) and their role in septic shock, substances were developed to quickly neutralize them. At the same time, the relationships between disease activity of rheumatoid arthritis (RA) and IL-1 and TNF-α were becoming better understood [125]. Technological advances in the production of humanized monoclonal antibodies and initial good experiences in the therapy of rheumatoid arthritis (RA) with anti-CD4 antibodies paved the way for long-term treatment of RA and other chronic inflammatory diseases with IL-1/TNF-α binding substances [97].

Clinical Aspects

Anemias of Rheumatoid Arthritis

Due to a chronic inflammatory process, rheumatoid arthritis (RA) leads to the gradual, progressive destruction of joint cartilage and bone. The disease is not limited to joints, however. It is also frequently manifested in other organs such as the heart, eyes, and kidneys.

In every case, the joints become inflamed. This inflammation is accompanied by a strong, painful swelling of the synovial membrane (Fig. 36). Connective tissue then proliferates in the cartilage, which eventually destroys the joint cartilage and the exposed bone. In the cases of pronounced activity, the patient also suffers from anemia and thrombocytosis.

Neutrophils accumulate in the synovial fluid, while macrophages and T-lymphocytes in particular accumulate in the synovial membrane. Cell infiltration and the regeneration of blood vessels cause the synovial membrane to thicken (formation of pannus). During this process, large quantities of macrophages are located in the border of the synovial membrane and in the cartilage contact zone. The macrophages and fibroblasts are induced via proinflammatory cytokines (e.g., TNF-α and IL-1) to release collagenase and stromelysin 1, two matrix metalloproteinases that play a significant role in the destruction of cartilage. Osteoclasts are stimulated (Figs. 35, 36).

The laboratory findings in patients with rheumatoid arthritis are depicted in Table 29.

Table 29: Laboratory diagnostics of rheumatoid diseases

	CRP	RF	ASL, ADNase	ANA	CCP-AB
Rheumatoid arthritis	++	++	–	+	++
Rheumatic fever	+	(+)	++	(+)	–
Collagenoses, e.g. SLE	(+)	(+)	–	+++	–

CRP: C-reactive protein
RF: Rheumatoid Factor
ASL: Antistreptolysin titer
ADNase: Streptodornase
ANA: Antinuclear antibodies
SLE: Systemic lupus erythematodes
CCP-AB: Antibodies against cyclic citrullinated proteins

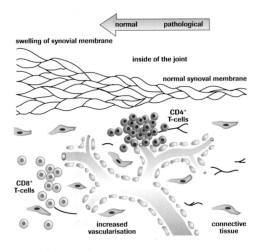

Fig. 36: Cell structure of the synovialis

Excess quantities of released tumor necrosis factor alpha (TNF-α) – which are secreted by activated monocytes, macrophages and dendritic cells, and IL-1, the main task of which is macrophage activation – play a central role in the induction of rheumatoid arthritis. Both cytokines suppress via activation of interferon (IFN) the formation of CFU-E (col-

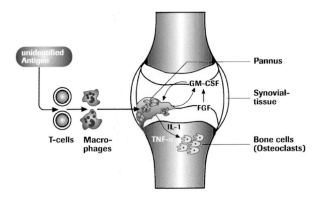

Fig. 37: Induction of rheumatic arthritis (according to Ref. [30])
    FGF, Fibroblast growth factor; GM-CSF, granulocycle macrophage monocycte
    colony-stimulating factor

ony-forming unit – erythrocytic) and, depending on their concentration, they intervene massively in the erythropoietic maturation sequence and the biologic activity of erythropoietin. TNF-α and IL-1 (via IFN-γ) are antagonists of EPO. High concentrations of TNF-α and IL-1, due to the massive suppression of erythropoiesis, can lead to hypochromic anemia.

Erythropoietin and Iron Therapy of Rheumatoid Arthritis

Iron metabolism in monocytes/macrophages plays an especially significant role in chronic disease. The organism uses iron metabolism in the inflammatory and anti-neoplastic defense system. It draws iron from microorganisms and neoplastic cells and stores it in reticuloendothelial systems. This is characterized by the development of normochromic, normocytic or microcytic anemia (ACD = Anemias of Chronic Disease). This type of anemia is caused by all types of inflammation (rheumatoid arthritis, malignant growths, or trauma). Due to various cytokines (TNF-α, IL1, IL-6, and IFN-γ), erythropoiesis is compromised primarily at the CFU-E level in this process.

Iron and erythropoietin therapy in patients with chronic inflammation can be assessed as promising [36, 106], as in addition to improving the anemia, the previously described inhibiting effect of iron on cytokine action and macrophage-induced cytotoxicity has a favorable influence.

As under erythropoietin administration the transferrin receptor on erythroid precursor cells is upregulated the sequential administration of erythropoietin and iron (at intervals of 48 hours) should be discussed [149, 150].

Concomitant anemia, which is severe and also microcytic in some cases, can be successfully treated by erythropoietin substitution [69]. The patients were treated with 150 IU rhu-EPO per kg body weight twice weekly over a period of 12 weeks. Where there was a functional iron deficit, the patients were additionally given 200 mg Fe^{3+}-sucrose weekly i.v.

All patients showed normalization of Hb concentration and quality of life as measured by various parameters such as multi-dimensional assessment of fatigue (MAF) and muscle strength index (MSI). Laboratory parameters for the activity of rheumatoid arthritis (RA) and rheumatoid arthritis disease activity index (RADAI) also showed a clear improvement during erythropoietin therapy. Upon cessation of therapy after the 12-week period there was – as expected – a decrease in the improvement achieved.

In order to achieve optimum management of patients treated with rhu-EPO in combination with intravenous iron injections, the iron balance parameters should be determined at regular intervals (Table 30). At the moment, virtually identical recommendations apply to both the treatment of anemia in RA (iron distribution disorder) and anemia due to renal failure (erythropoietin deficiency and iron utilization disorder).

Table 30: Recommendations for patients receiving EPO/i.v. iron therapy. EPO: 3 × 50 or 1 × 150 IU/kg/week; i.v. iron: 10–40 (correction) or 10–20 (monitoring) mg/week

Diagnostic parameter	Target values	Frequency of determination
Hemoglobin (g/dL)	12	Every 3 months
Hematocrit (%)	30–36	
Reticulocyte production index (RPI)	>2	
Folate (µg/L)	>20	Every 6 months
Vitamin B$_{12}$ (µg/L)	>2	
Ferritin (µg/L)	100–300	At the beginning of correction phase and every three months after the end of correction phase
sTfR (mg/L)	<5	
TfS (%)	>15 (monitoring: 15–45)	
Hypochromic erythrocytes (%)	<10	
CRP (mg/L)	<5mg/L (monitoring)	

Clinical Aspects

Disturbances of Iron Utilization

In patients with disturbances of iron utilization, the individual erythrocyte contains a normal amount of hemoglobin despite the lowering of the patient's hemoglobin value. MCH and MCV are normal. Iron deficiency is apparently not the problem in this case, but rather the erythrocyte balance between formation and decomposition. This balance is reflected in the reticulocyte count (as a measure of the regeneration of erythropoiesis) with normal reticulocyte values between 5 and 15‰.

- Normochromic and normoregenerative anemias are usually based on inadequate stimulation of erythropoiesis. In patients with renal anemia, erythropoietin synthesis is greatly reduced when chronic renal insufficiency is present.
- Increased reticulocyte production index values >2 are measured in patients with hyperregeneration. It is the response to the increased decomposition of erythrocytes by hemolysis. When erythrocyte decomposition is elevated, haptoglobin is used as the transport protein for hemoglobin and it drops rapidly. Haptoglobin is therefore a marker for the diagnosis of hemolysis. Bilirubin increases noticeably only in the presence of acute or relatively intense erythrocyte decomposition.
- Lowered reticulocyte production index values <2 are measured primarily in the presence of hyporegeneration, i.e., hypoplasia or even aplasia in the bone marrow, or in deficiency anemias.

Uremic Anemia

Uremic anemia is an important special form of normochromic normocytic anemia. The clinical finding that plasma erythropoietin is lower in uremic patients than in non-uremic patients with a comparable degree of anemia suggests that uremic anemia is caused by the inadequate production of erythropoietin in renal failure.

Although uremic anemia is obviously multifactorial in origin and can be partially improved by appropriate hemodialysis therapy, the role played by the extracorporeal hemolytic component must not be underestimated. Many patients have developed a defect in the hexose mono-

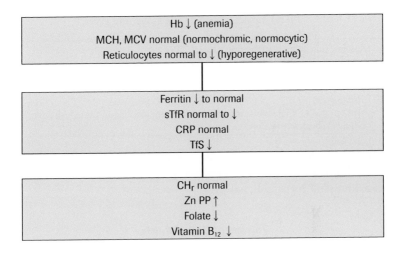

sTfR   =   soluble transferrin receptor
TfS   =   Transferrin saturation
CRP   =   C-reactive protein
CH$_r$ =   hemoglobin content of reticulocytes
Zn PP =   zinc protoporphyrin

Fig. 38: Laboratory findings in patients with uremic anemia without EPO therapy or transfusion

phosphate shunt; in addition, influences in hemodialysis such as mechanical intravascular hemolysis or pump trauma play an increasing role.

The concentrations of the soluble transferrin receptors in plasma are lower in these patients than in healthy subjects even when the ferritin depots are adequate [51].

This is not surprising if we bear in mind that the main production centers of the transferrin receptor are the immature cells of erythropoiesis, which are reduced in mass in chronic renal failure. Therefore it would appear that soluble transferrin receptor production in renal anemias is dependent on erythropoietin.

Remarkably, uremic anemia is well tolerated by patients and hemoglobin values down to 5 g/dL are well tolerated without side-effects. In most patients, the reticulocyte count is low and the survival time of blood cells is only moderately decreased. Anemia is thus the result of a massively disturbed erythrocyte production in the bone marrow.

Clinical Aspects

Table 31: Causes of reduced response to rhu-EPO in patients with renal anemia

- Absolute iron deficiency (ferritin < 100 µg/L, TfS < 20%)
- Functional iron deficiency (ferritin > 100 µg/L, TfS < 20%)
- Chronic blood losses
- Infection and inflammation (leukocytes and CRP)
- Malignancies
- Medications (ACE inhibitors, angiotensin II receptor blocking agents in high doses, cyclophosphamide, azathioprin)

If there are adequate ferritin depots, uremic anemia can be slightly improved by hemodialysis. A successful kidney transplant is the only way to achieve full correction, however.

Therapy of Uremic Anemia

Possible causes of inadequate response to rhEPO are listed in Table 31. If functional iron deficiency exists, determination of the hypochromic erythrocytes (or reticulocyte Hb) is often helpful. If the portion of this erythrocyte subpopulation is above 10%, parenteral iron substitution will definitely improve the response of erythropoiesis to rhu-EPO. About 150 mg iron is required to raise hemoglobin by 1 g/dL. In order to correct hemoglobin by 3–4 g/dL, therefore, 450–600 mg iron is required for hemoglobin synthesis. Hemolysis patients require increased doses of iron, e.g., about 2–3 g per year, for the duration of erythropoietin treatment due to the loss of blood incurred in the course of treatment. Such amounts of iron typically must be administered parenterally, as the majority of patients do not tolerate higher doses of oral iron therapy due to intestinal side-effects. The risk of an iatrogenic iron overload during long-term replacement with parenteral iron is minimal as long as ferritin is monitored regularly.

Anaphylactoidal reactions of the type described in the context of ferric dextran – still widely used in the United States – are rare occurrences when Ferrlecit® or Venofer® is used [73].

Patients with chronic renal insufficiency, including those on chronic hemodialysis (CHD) and frequent blood transfusions are favorite candidates for rhEPO therapy.

The rapidity and extent of the hematocrit increase can be regulated by the rhEPO dose. Poor response may be caused by iron deficiency due to inadequate iron stores or deficient iron mobilization from these stores (functional iron deficiency). An increasing hypochromia of erythrocytes and reticulocytes is often an early indicator of this.

Further causes of a diminished ability to respond to rhEPO are vitamin B_{12} and folic acid deficiency or a reduction in stem cells in the bone marrow of patients with secondary hyperparathyroidism.

The difficulty to be mastered with the therapy of renal anemia is to correct the transport iron deficiency and concomitanly avoid a significant iron overload. Absolute or functional iron deficiency can be excluded if the transferrin saturation is significantly higher than 20% and ferritin level exceeds 100 µg/L.

Low serum ferritin values (less than 100 µg/L) in patients with uremia signify an absolute iron deficiency. High ferritin values, however, do not completely exclude functional iron deficiency.

Functional iron deficiency is characterized by normal (100–400 µg/L) or elevated (above 400 µg/L) ferritin values as well as reduced transferrin saturation values (less than 20%) and elevated sTfR values.

Criteria for a sufficient supply of iron are a ferritin level of at least 100 µg/L and a transferrin saturation of more than 20%. The soluble transferrin receptor concentration should be less than 5 mg/L (values are dependent on the method used) [83].

If dialysis patients do not meet these criteria, 10 mg of iron per dialysis should be administered after replenishing the iron depot to a ferritin level of 100 µg/L. In non-dialysis patients oral iron replacement may be adequate (100–300 mg/day of iron(II)).

The therapeutic aim is to increase the hemoglobin concentration to 11–13 g/dL. The total average iron requirement of an adult can be estimated using the following simple formula [72]:

Iron requirement (mg) = 150 mg × (Hb1 – Hb0)

Hb0: initial hemoglobin concentration.
Hb1: target hemoglobin concentration.

This formula provides a good estimation. For cases of extreme anemia or iron deficiency, however, the use of Cook's equation is recommended (see below). The target values for the various parameters are listed in Table 32.

Clinical Aspects

Table 32: Recommendations for EPO and iron treatment of dialysis patients and targets for the different parameters of iron metabolism

	Correction		Maintenance of Hb (ferritin) concentration
EPO: About 2000 IU/patient/dialysis with 3 dialyses per week			
i.v. iron:	10–40 mg/week	i.v. iron:	10–20 mg/week
Hb:	10–12 g/dL	Hb:	11–13 g/dL
Ferritin:	100 µg/L	Ferritin:	<400 µg/L
TfS:	15–45%	TfS:	15–45%
sTfR:	<5 mg/L	sTfR:	<5 mg/L
CRP:	<5 mg/L	CRP:	<5 mg/L

Ferritin concentrations of over 400 µg/L should be avoided in the long term on account of the concomitant danger of iron deposits forming outside the reticuloendothelial system. If values exceed this threshold during intravenous therapy, then a break in the therapy for a period of 3 months should be considered but erythropoietin treatment should be continued. The danger of iron overload in the context of parenteral substitution therapy adapted to iron losses of approximately 1.0–1.5 g per year can be considered to be low for hemodialysis patients. In the maintenance phase a low-dose, high-frequency administration of iron (10 to a maximum of 20 mg iron saccharate per hemodialysis) is currently preferred.

As demonstrated by the results of determining CRP, IL-6 (interleukin-6), orosomucoid (alpha-1-acid-glycoprotein), and SAA (serum amyloid A), no acute phase reaction occurred in patients undergoing dialysis and receiving iron. Possible side-effects of long-term iron supplementation leading to ferritin values >400 µg/L are: increased risk of infection, elevated risk of developing carcinomas, and an increased cardiovascular risk [110, 135]. Iron overload should be avoided during rhu-EPO therapy with concomitant iron supplementation.

In the context of the therapy of uremic anemia, the erythropoietin doses administered should be matched to the individual needs of the patient because the amount required by the uremic patient can be subject to considerable change. The dose can be significantly reduced in

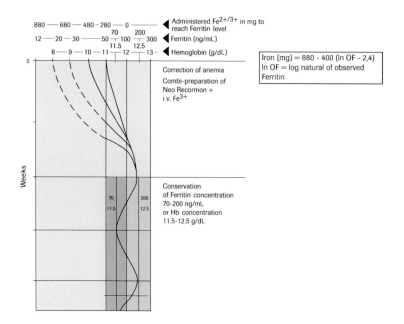

Fig. 39: Nomogram for the determination of the amount of iron required to achieve target values of 100 µg/L ferritin and 12 g/dL hemoglobin while maintaining administration of EPO constant

dialysis patients receiving optimized intravenous iron therapy. Hörl et al. reported a reduction in the mean EPO dosage from 220 to 60 U/kg/week and a reduction from 140 to 70 U/kg/week [72].

The often discussed question of whether the dosage of erythropoietin is influenced by the route of administration is best answered by pointing out that, on parenteral iron therapy, there is no significant difference in the amount of erythropoietin required by intravenous and by subcutaneous administration. Similar observations were made by Hörl et al. [72] and Sunder-Plasmann [136].

Cook et al. [38] as well as Mercuriali et al. [104] developed a therapeutic regimen for hemodialysis patients receiving rhu-EPO in which the targets are 100 µg/L serum ferritin and a transferrin saturation of more than 20% in order to ensure provision of adequate amounts of iron without the risk of iron overload. The required iron doses can be calculated using the following formula:

i.v. iron (mg) = 880 – 400 × (ln OF – 2.4)
   OF = Observed ferritin
   ln OF = ln of observed ferritin

2.4 = ln of serum ferritin value of 12 μg/L
Example:
Observed serum ferritin value OF = 50 μg/L
   ln OF = 3.9

i.v. iron amount (mg) = 880 – 400 × (3.9 – 2.4) = 880 – 400 × 1.5 = 280 mg

That means, 280 mg of i.v. iron are required to increase the ferritin level of the dialysis patient from 50 μg/L to 100 μg/L. This should be achieved in 10 dialysis sessions, i.e., within 3–4 weeks.

The amount of iron required to achieve target values of 100 μg/L ferritin and 12 g/dL hemoglobin can also be determined using the nomogram shown in Fig. 39.

Iron Overload

The human body is incapable of actively excreting excess iron. An overabundant supply of iron leads to increased concentrations of the iron storage proteins ferritin and hemosiderin. If the storage capacity is exceeded, deposition takes place in the parenchymatous organs. The resulting cell damage leads to cell death and to functional impairment of the organ in question.

It has been suggested that this damage is due to toxic effects of free iron ions on the enzyme metabolism and to lysosome damage.

Iron overload, unlike iron deficiency, is rare. However, it is often overlooked or misinterpreted, and can progress to a life-threatening stage as a result. An elevated ferritin level should always suggest an iron overload, and the possibility of a true iron overload should be explored by differential diagnosis (Fig. 40). On the other hand, disturbances of iron distribution must also be considered as a possibility (Table 33).

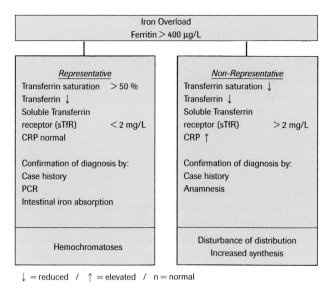

$\downarrow$ = reduced / $\uparrow$ = elevated / n = normal

Fig. 40: Differential diagnosis of clinical pictures with elevated ferritin levels

Table 33: Causes of iron overload

---

  1. Primary, hereditary hemochromatosis

  2. Secondary acquired hemochromatosis

     • Ineffective erythropoiesis

     – Thalassemia major

     – Sideroblastic anemias

     – Aplastic anemias

     • Transfusion

  3. Diet-related hemochromatosis

     • Excessive iron intake

     – Chronic alcoholism

HLA: human leukocyte antigen

Iron overload diseases can be divided into primary hereditary forms, and various secondary forms, or acquired hemochromatoses. The secondary forms are also known as hemosideroses.

Primary Hematochromatosis

Currently different mutations causing primary hematochromatosis are described:

- Type 1:   HFE – HFE protein
- Type 2A: HJV – Hemojuvelin
- Type 2B: HAMP – Hepcidin
- Type 3:   TFR2 – Transferrin Receptor 2
- Type 4:   SLC11A3 – Ferroportin

In more than 80% of the patients primary hemochromatosis is caused by gene mutations on the short arm of chromosome 6 (HFE gene). They lead to increased iron absorption in the small intestine and increased iron storage in the affected organs, namely the parenchymal cells of the liver, the heart, the pancreas, and the adrenal glands with the appropriate accompanying clinical complications such as diabetes, cirrhosis of the liver, arthropathy, cardiomyopathy, and impotence.

The HFE gene product – which is responsible for increased absorption of iron – is localized in the gastrointestinal tract and in the mutated form it is not capable of migrating out of the cell. The prevalence of the disease is between 4 and 14% in Europe with a significant divide between North and South.

Men are affected approximately 10 times more often than women by primary hemochromatosis which becomes clinically manifest between the ages of 35 and 55 and causes liver function disorders, diabetes mellitus, dark pigmentation of the skin, cardiomyopathy, and resulting arrhythmia. Furthermore, complaints of the joints and symptoms due to secondary hypogonadism as well as adrenal gland insufficiency have been observed. In about 15% of those affected by the illness, liver cell carcinoma arises, which represents a 300-fold risk.

In primary hemochromatosis, the plasma ferritin level rises at a relatively late stage. Initially parenchymal cells of the liver, heart, and pancreas as well as other organs are overloaded with iron and only thereafter is the reticuloendothelial system saturated. Ferritin values above 400 µg/L and a transferrin saturation of more than 50% signify existing iron overload. In the manifest stage of primary hemochromatosis, ferritin concentrations in serum are usually over 700 µg/L. Transferrin is almost completely saturated.

Liver biopsy was the most appropriate in the past to conclusively diagnose primary hyperchromatosis, but a major advance has been made recently by the advent of identifying specific genetic changes for diagnosing the disease. The genetic defect can be identified using a molecular biologic test. Hemochromatosis can be identified in 80% of the cases using the simple and relatively economically feasible PCR and DNA sequencing technologies before the manifestation of clinical symptoms. This opens up the possibility of timely treatment such that late-stage complications like cirrhosis of the liver and cancer of the liver can be prevented.

Phlebotomy is still of widespread use. The aim of the therapy is to deplete iron stores as much as possible. The determination of the body iron status should be performed frequently at short intervals and in hereditary hemochromatosis the determination of plasma ferritin has proven to be of worth. The progression of the clinical parameter determines the necessity of continuing phlebotomy therapy. Phlebotomy at weekly, monthly or quarterly intervals may be necessary; however, the therapy should never completely cease. As described above, the aim of phlebotomy is to prevent a negative progression of the disease.

Clinical Aspects

Early identification of patients at risk which has become possible by virtue of the molecular biologic detection of genetic defects can probably drastically reduce the incidence of hepatocellular carcinomas. Careful monitoring is required using imaging procedures (sonography, computer tomography [CT], nuclear magnetic resonance [NMR]), and regular determination of the α-fetoprotein (AFP).

Secondary Hemochromatosis

Hematopoietic disorders with concomitant ineffective or hypoplastic erythropoiesis such as thalassemia major, sideroblastic anemia or aplastic anemia are considered to be secondary or acquired hemochromatoses. In contrast to primary hemochromatosis in the secondary form the cells of the reticuloendothelial system are initially overloaded with iron. Organ damage occurs at a relatively late stage. They arise because of a redistribution of iron from the cells of the reticuloendothelial system into parenchymal cells of individual organs. The duration of chronic iron overloading in secondary iron storage disorders is therefore a critical factor.

Acquired hemochromatoses can also develop from alimentary iron overload, parenteral administration of iron, and transfusions or other chronic diseases with ineffective erythrocytopoiesis.

Alcoholics with chronic liver disease in whom iron deposits have been detected after liver biopsies but whose total body iron levels are within the non-pathologic range present a particular diagnostic challenge. The body's total iron reserves are normal. Such patients probably suffer from an alcohol-induced liver disease (toxic nutritive cirrhosis) and seem to acquire iron deposits as a result of cell necroses and iron uptake from such necrotic cells.

However, a second group of alcoholics has been identified who have extremely high deposits of iron in their bodies and massive iron deposits in the cirrhotic liver. Such patients may suffer from congenital primary hemochromatosis with concomitant toxic nutritive liver disease. The molecular biologic detection of causative primary hemochromatosis makes differential diagnosis more straightforward.

Patients suffering from renal insufficiency on dialysis were first treated with erythropoietin in 1988 and for this group of patients, iron overloading caused by transfusions should belong firmly to the past.

Non-iron-induced Disturbances of Erythropoiesis

Deficiencies in vitamin B_{12}, folic acid and/or erythropoietin have been found to be crucial factors in non-iron-deficiency-induced forms of anemia.

An initial diagnosis can be made with a high degree of accuracy by recording the patient's history or from knowledge of the primary disease. Given the known interaction between vitamin B_{12} and folic acid, the determination of these two cofactors by immunoassay should now be standard clinical practice. Sternal puncture or bone biopsies also offer clear histologic and morphologic pictures.

Deficiency in folic acid or vitamin B_{12} is the main feature of diseases accompanied by macrocytic anemia.

In the differential diagnosis of macrocytic anemia, an elevated level of LDH with simultaneous reticulocytosis and hyperbilirubinemia (both to be interpreted as hyperregeneratory anemia) directs attention to a vitamin B_{12} deficit. Macrocytic anemia without these components makes a genuine folic acid deficiency likely (pregnancy and alcohol).

Normocytic forms of anemia draw attention to the hemolytic component of erythrocyte destruction, with haptoglobin playing the crucial role as the key to diagnosis. Erythrocyte morphology provides a means to exclude mechanical hemolysis or to look for hemoglobinopathy (Hb electrophoresis) or an enzyme defect.

Proof of impaired renal function makes it likely that a deficiency of erythropoietin is present.

Table 34: Deficiencies in the cofactors of erythropoiesis

Microcytic anemia	Macrocytic anemia	Normocytic anemia
Iron metabolism disturbances Hemoglobinopathies (e.g., thalassemia)	Folic acid deficiency B_{12} deficiency Drug-induced Alcohol consumption MDS	Renal anemia (erythropoietin deficiency) Hemolytic anemia Hemoglobinopathies Bone marrow diseases Toxic bone marrow damage

MDS: Myelodysplastic syndrome

The determination of erythropoietin which is performed by immu-noassay at least forms a good base for the prognosis of the outcome of treatment. Before giving any treatment with erythropoietin, it is impor-tant to determine the iron depots; otherwise, action by the parenterally administered erythropoietin, which is genetically engineered today, is impossible.

Macrocytic, Hyperchromic Anemia

Hyperchromic macrocytic anemias (MCH above 33 pg, MCV usually above 96 fL) and a typical blood count almost always indicate a vitamin deficiency of B_6, B_{12} or folic acid and normo- to hyporegeneratory (RPI below 2). In advanced stages, vitamin deficiency can also affect the re-

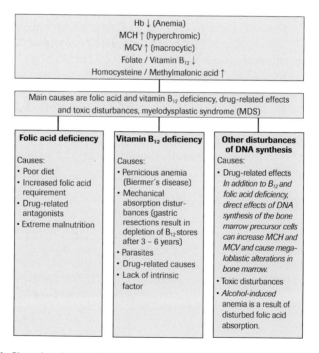

Fig. 41: Diagnosis and causes of macrocytic, hyperchromic anemias

maining cell lines (leukocytopenia and thrombocytopenia). The most frequent cause of a hyperchromic anemia is chronic alcoholism (Fig. 41).

A non-representative ferritin increase may indicate disturbances in the proliferation and maturation of bone marrow cells induced by vitamin deficiency.

These macrocytic forms of anemia are caused by disturbed DNA synthesis. As non-iron-induced disturbances of erythropoiesis, they influence not only the proliferation of cells of erythropoiesis, but above all that of the gastrointestinal epithelial cells. Since considerable numbers of macrocytic cells are destroyed while still in the bone marrow, they are also included under the heading ineffective erythropoiesis.

Most macrocytic forms of anemia are due to a deficiency in either vitamin B_{12} or folic acid, or both. The most common causes of macrocytic anemia are listed in Tables 35 and 36.

Table 35: Drug-induced forms of macrocytic anemia

Drugs which act via folic acid malabsorption
- Alcohol, phenytoin, and barbiturates

Drugs which act via folic acid metabolism
- Alcohol, methotrexate, pyrimethamine, triamterene, and pentamidine

Drugs which act via vitamin B_{12}
- PAS, colchicine, and neomycin

Inhibitors of nucleic acid metabolism
- Purine antagonists (azathioprine and 6-mercaptopurine)
- Pyrimidine antagonists (5-fluorouracil, and cytosine arabinoside)
- Others (procarbazine, aciclovir, zidovudine, and hydroxyurea)

PAS = para-aminosalicylic acid

Table 36: Symptomatic forms of macrocytic anemia

Metabolic diseases
- Aciduria (orotic acid)

Uncertain origin
- Di Guglielmo syndrome
- Congenital dyserthopoietic anemia
- Refractory megaloblastic anemia

Clinical Aspects

Drug-induced macrocytic anemia is now common. Drugs which disturb DNA synthesis are now part of the standard therapeutic armamentarium of chemotherapy (Table 35). There are also rare metabolic disturbances which cause macrocytic anemia, plus megaloblastic anemia with as yet unknown causes, such as the congenital dyserythropoietic anemias or anemias as part of the Di Guglielmo syndrome (Table 36).

Acute severe macrocytic anemia is a rarity; it can be observed in intensive care patients who require multiple transfusions, hemodialysis or total parenteral nutrition. This form of acute macrocytic anemia may be limited mainly to patients who already had borderline folic acid depots before they fell ill.

Folic Acid

Folic acid is reduced to tetrahydrofolic acid (THF) in the organism under the influence of ascorbic acid and vitamin B_{12}. As a transporter of activated C-1 groups (methyl-, formyl-, formiate-, and hydroxymethyl groups), tetrahydrofolic acid performs an important function in amino acid and nucleotide metabolism and in the methylation of homocysteine to methionine. Folic acid is essential for the biosynthesis of purines and pyrimidines for DNA and RNA synthesis and, therefore, for all growth and cellular division processes. Since the erythropoietic cells of the bone marrow have high rates of cellular division, they are particularly dependent on an adequate supply of folic acid. A schematic overview of folic acid, vitamin B_{12}, and vitamin B_6 metabolism is given by Fig. 17.

The body's total folic acid reserves are approximately 5–10 mg. The German Society for Nutrition recommends a daily intake of 400 mg folic acid (dietary folate). The recommendation for women who are pregnant or breast-feeding is 600 mg folic acid (dietary folate) per day.

Due to the poor dietary intake of folic acid by the United States population, certain basic foodstuffs (breakfast cereals and flour) have been enriched with folic acid in the United States since 1998.

The National Research Council of the United States recommends a daily dietary allowance of folic acid of 400 mg for adults up to 55 years of age. For adults above 55 years of age, the recommended dietary allowance (RDA) is 800–1200 mg/day.

Table 37: Causes of folic acid deficiency

---

1. Inadequate intake
   – Alcoholism
   – Unbalanced diet
2. Increased requirement
   – Pregnancy
   – Adolescence
   – Malignancy
   Increased cell turnover (hemolysis and chronic exfoliative skin diseases)
   Hemodialysis patients
3. Malabsorption
   – Sprue
   – Drugs (barbiturates and phenytoin)
4. Disturbed folic acid metabolism
   – Inhibition of dihydrofolic acid reductase (e.g., methotrexate,
     pyrimethamin, and triamterene)
   – Congenital enzyme defects

Patients with a folic acid deficit are usually in a poor nutritional state, and often have a range of gastrointestinal symptoms such as diarrhea, cheilosis, and glossitis. In contrast to advanced vitamin B_{12} deficiency, no neurologic deficits are found.

Folic acid deficiency can be attributed to three main causes: inadequate intake, increased requirement, and malabsorption (Table 37).

Special attention must be devoted to various groups in the population who commonly have inadequate folic acid intake: chronic alcoholics, the elderly, and adolescents.

In chronic alcoholics, alcoholic beverages are the main source of energy which contain at most small quantities of folic acid.

Alcohol also leads to disturbances in the processing of absorbed folic acid.

The folic acid deficit in the elderly seems to be caused mainly by an extremely unbalanced diet.

Unbalanced diets have a considerable attraction for adolescents. Those who consume fast food are particularly at risk.

An increased folic acid requirement is present during the growth phase in childhood and adolescence, as well as during pregnancy.

Since the bone marrow and the intestinal mucosa have an increased folic acid requirement because of a high cell proliferation rate, patients

Clinical Aspects

with hematologic diseases, especially those with increased erythropoiesis, may not be able to meet their increased folic acid requirement from their dietary intake.

Disturbances in the absorption of folic acid occur in both tropical sprue and gluten enteropathy. Manifest macrocytic anemia may develop in both clinical pictures. Other signs of malabsorption may also occur. Alcohol-induced folic acid deficiency may to a certain extent also be caused by malabsorption. Diseases of the small intestine may also prevent the absorption of folic acid.

The folic acid absorption test is used as a general, practical means for detecting malabsorption. For this test the patient is given 1 mg folic acid i.v. or i.m. per day on the 4 days preceding the examination. This serves to make up any folic acid deficiency in the tissue which could affect the absorption test and produce a false positive result (no measurable increase in the serum folic acid concentration after oral ingestion). On the day of the examination the fasting patient is given 40 mg/kg folic acid orally, and the serum folic acid concentration is determined at the following times: 0, 60, and 120 minutes. In normal patients the serum concentration rises to over 7 mg/L.

Folic acid is absorbed in the entire small intestine, so that the substance is suitable for a test of small-intestine absorption. Data on normal serum concentrations vary from laboratory to laboratory, but do not diverge to any great extent [44]. Findings by Brouwer [27], however, suggest that the currently used reference range should be corrected.

Low levels of folic acid in the serum or in the erythrocytes are a definite indication of folic acid deficiency. This condition is treated by oral replacement therapy, with 1 mg folic acid being administered daily. The reaction to the replacement therapy is similar to that in B_{12} deficiency, i.e. within 5–7 days there is an increase in the number of reticulocytes and the blood count returns to normal within 2–3 months.

Due to the disturbed development of erythrocyte, a deficiency of folic acid or vitamin B_{12} can lead to the formation of a macrocytic or megaloblastic anemia. Cell division in the erythropoietic cells in the bone marrow is slowed, so that megalocytes, instead of normal erythrocytes (normocytes), are formed. Megalocytes contain too much hemoglobin as compared to normal red blood cells.

To prevent neural tube defects, women who desire to become pregnant are recommended to begin early replacement of 0.4–0.8 mg folic acid per day.

Folic acid replacement can mask a deficiency of vitamin B_{12} (secondary folic acid deficiency in patients with pernicious anemia). Vitamin B_{12} returns N-methyl-tetrahydrofolic acid to tetrahydrofolic acid, which is important for DNA synthesis. Although inhibition of this conversion by vitamin B_{12} deficiency can be compensated by administering folic acid, the danger of severe neurologic damage remains. The main cause of folic acid deficiency is an inadequate supply in the food (alcoholism, unbalanced diets, and drugs). If these factors are not present in the patient's history, a B_{12} deficiency should also be ruled out.

Vitamin B$_{12}$

Cobalamin contained in food is taken up as methyl-cobalamin, hydroxy-cobalamin, and deoxyadenosyl-cobalamin. In the acid environment of the stomach cobalamin is released from the food proteins bound to the R-protein which is produced by the salivary glands and is present in the gastric juice. Cobalamin has a severalfold higher affinity to R-protein than to intrinsic factor.

In the duodenum, given a neutral pH, the R-protein is broken down by pancreatic peptidases and cobalamin is released. The latter now binds to intrinsic factor and the intrinsic factor-cobalamin complex moves on to the ileum. Once there, the complex binds to a specific receptor of the mucosal cell. Cobalamin is absorbed, reaches the portal venous blood, and then a portion of it binds to transcobalamin II which is synthesized by the endothelial cells of the blood vessels. The major portion of cobalamin, however, is bound to transcobalamins I and III; both of these proteins are synthesized by granulocytes. However, the tissue only takes up cobalamin bound to transcobalamin II. In the cells, cobalamin II is transformed into its active forms (5′-deoxyadenosyl-cobalamin and methylcobalamin).

These substances are involved in the biosynthesis of purine and pyrimidine bases, the synthesis of methionine from homocysteine, in the regeneration of N-methyl-tetrahydrofolic acid (secondary folic acid deficiency in patients with pernicious anemia) and the formation of my-

Clinical Aspects

elin sheaths in the nervous system. Vitamin B_{12}, as well as folic acid, is involved in DNA synthesis and, consequently, has a strong influence on all cell division and growth processes (Fig. 41).

The symptoms of vitamin B_{12} deficiency are partly hematologic, partly gastroenterologic. Neurologic manifestations are often observed independently of the duration of vitamin B_{12} deficiency.

Table 38: Causes of vitamin B_{12} deficiency

Inadequate intake
- – Vegetarians (rare)

Malabsorption
- Deficiency of intrinsic factor
  – Pernicious anemia
  – Gastrectomy
  – Congenital (extremely rare)
- Diseases of the terminal ileum
  – Sprue
  – Crohn's disease
  – Extensive resections
  – Selective malabsorption (Imerslund syndrome – extremely rare)
- Parasite-induced deficiencies
  – Fish tapeworm
  – Bacteria ("blind loop syndrome")
- Drug-induced
  – PAS, neomycin

PAS: paraaminosalicylic acid

The hematologic symptoms are almost always caused by an anemia. They include paleness, weakness, dizziness, tinnitus as well as coronary heart disease, and myocardial insufficiency.

There is usually tachycardia with an enlarged heart; the liver and spleen may also be slightly enlarged. Fissures in the mucous membrane, a red tongue, anorexia, weight loss, and occasional diarrhea indicate that the gastrointestinal system is involved.

It may be very difficult to classify the neurologic symptoms. Irrespective of the duration of the vitamin B_{12} deficit, in extreme cases they may range from demyelinization to neuron death. The earliest neurologic manifestations consist of paresthesia, weakness, ataxia, and disturbances of fine coordination. Objectively, disturbance of deep sensibility usually occurs early and *Rhomberg and Babinski* are positive. The CNS symptoms range from forgetfulness to severe forms of dementia or psychoses. These neurologic conditions may long precede the hematologic manifestations, but as a rule hematologic symptoms predominate in the average patient.

The main cause of vitamin B_{12} deficiency, the pernicious anemia, is a deficiency of intrinsic factor. It is generally accompanied by atrophy of the gastric mucosa.

Vitamin B_{12} deficiency shows geographical clustering in Northern Europe. It is generally a disease affecting the elderly beyond the age of 60; it is less common in children younger than 10 years old. It is found with striking frequency in black patients.

The current view about the pathogenesis of pernicious anemia is that it is produced by an autoimmune process directed against the parietal cells of the stomach. It is therefore most marked in patients with clinical pictures attributed to autoimmune diseases, such as immune hyperthyroidism, myxedema, idiopathic adrenal insufficiency, vitiligo, and hypoparathyroidism. Antibodies against parietal cells can be detected in 90% of patients with pernicious anemia. The detection of these antibodies does not however mean that the pernicious anemia is necessarily manifest. The incidence of antibodies to intrinsic factor is about 60%.

Given the pathologic mechanism involved, hypoacidity or anacidity is the rule, patients often have gastric polyps, and the incidence of stomach cancer doubles that in the normal population. If the source of the intrinsic factor is destroyed such as by total gastrectomy or by extensive destruction of the gastric mucosa (for example by corrosion) megaloblastic anemia may develop.

It should also not be forgotten that a number of bacteria in the intestinal flora require vitamin B_{12}. Deficiency syndromes may thus develop after anatomical lesions as a result of massive bacterial proliferation. Deficiency symptoms may also occur as a result of strictures, diverticula, and the blind loop syndrome. They may also occur with pseudo-obstruction in diabetes mellitus as a result of amyloid deposits, or in scleroderma. Vitamin B_{12}-deficiency anemia is also known to occur as a result of tropical sprue and the fish tapeworm. Most of these clinical pictures are also accompanied by malabsorption syndromes, often with steatorrhea.

Regional enteritis, Whipple's disease and tuberculosis may be accompanied by disturbances of vitamin B_{12} absorption. This also applies to chronic pancreatitis, in rare instances to Zollinger-Ellison syndrome, and segmental diseases of the ileum.

Defects of absorption of vitamin B_{12} used to be detected by the Schilling test. This test has been replaced by the determination of parietal cell antibodies and antibodies against intrinsic factor.

Hereditary megaloblastic anemia is extremely rare; it is caused by congenital disturbances of orotic acid metabolism or, in Lesch-Nyhan syndrome, by the disturbance of enzymes involved in folic acid metabolism.

The most frequent cause of B_{12} deficiency is a lack of intrinsic factor, as in pernicious anemia or after a total gastrectomy. Reduced absorption in the ileum after extensive surgical resection or in Crohn's disease may also be a cause. All other causes have little practical relevance. Vitamin B_{12} must therefore be administered parenterally.

On account of the neurologic and neuropsychiatric syndromes, which may also occur without blood count changes, and which are only then are definitely reversible if they have been present for less than 6 months, an initial high-dose treatment regimen has been established. This is a stepped regimen, in which 200 µg vitamin B_{12} is administered intramuscularly daily during the first week of therapy, followed by one intramuscular injection per week for 1 month and then monthly i.m. administration of 200 µg for the rest of the patient's life. It should be pointed out again that pernicious anemia is a life-long disease and that if the monthly treatment is interrupted, inevitably a vitamin deficiency will develop.

Clinical improvement is usually seen immediately after the administration of vitamin B_{12}. Between the 5th and 7th day, if there are sufficient iron reserves, the so-called reticulocytic crisis appears and within 2 months the peripheral blood count returns to normal. The CNS symptoms and their neurologic manifestations return to normal as well.

Normochromic, Normocytic Anemia

If the individual erythrocyte contains a normal amount of hemoglobin (MCH 28–33 pg/cell) despite the lowering of the patient's hemoglobin value, then iron deficiency is apparently not the problem in this case, but rather the erythrocyte balance between formation and decomposition. This balance is reflected in the reticulocyte count:

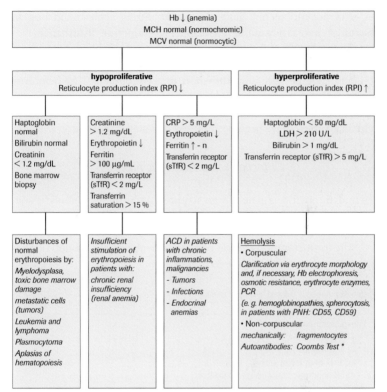

Fig. 42: Diagnosis and causes of normochromic, normocytic anemia

- Increased reticulocyte counts (>15%) are measured in patients with hyperregeneration. It is the response to the increased decomposition of erythrocytes (hemolysis).
- Lowered reticulocyte counts are measured primarily in the presence of hyporegeneration, i.e., hypoplasia or even aplasia in the bone marrow.
- When erythrocyte decomposition is elevated, haptoglobin is used as the transport protein for hemoglobin and it drops rapidly. Haptoglobin is therefore a marker for hemolysis. Bilirubin increases noticeably only in the presence of acute or relatively intense erythrocyte decomposition (hemolysis). Normal haptoglobin values indicate the absence of hemolysis.

Normocytic anemia generally occurs during acute blood loss, in hemolysis and as a result of renal failure or endocrine disturbances.

Besides the formal pathologic classification of anemia into microcytic, macrocytic and normocytic, differentiation by origin has now become established, especially in disturbances of erythropoiesis. The hemolytic anemias (cell trauma and membrane abnormality), enzyme disturbances (glucose-6-phosphate-dehydrogenase defect), and disturbances of hemoglobin synthesis have become clinically the most important.

Extracorpuscular Hemolytic Anemias

Hemolytic anemia is generally an acquired autoimmune hemolytic anemia. A common form of differentiation is based on the thermal behavior of the antibodies, as warm or cold antibodies.

The most common clinical pictures of symptomatic hemolytic anemia are summarized in Table 39.

Table 39: Antibody-induced hemolytic anemia

Warm antibodies
- Idiopathic
- Lymphomas
- Other neoplasms (rare)
- SLE (systemic lupus erythrematodes)
- Drugs

Cold antibodies
- Cold agglutinins

Infections (generally acute)

Lymphoma

Idiopathic
- Paroxysmal cold hemoglobinuria

Alloantibodies
- Blood transfusions

Pregnancies

In the detection of hemolysis, the determination of haptoglobin and LDH in particular has proved to be diagnostically useful test. After the occurrence of intravascular hemolysis, the serum haptoglobin concentration drops rapidly. This is attributable to the very short half-life of the haptoglobin-hemoglobin complex of only about 8 minutes. In its function as a transport (and acute-phase) protein it binds free hemoglobin and transports it extremely rapidly to the reticuloendothelial system for degradation.

Haptoglobin is therefore well suited for the diagnosis and assessment of the course of hemolytic diseases. Sharply decreased haptoglobin levels indicate intravascular hemolysis which may have immunohemolytic, microangiopathic, mechanical, drug (G-6-P-dehydrogenase deficiency) or infectious causes (e.g., malaria). Extravascular hemolysis (e.g., ineffective erythropoiesis and hypersplenism), on the other hand, shows a drop in haptoglobin only in hemolytic crises. Reduced haptoglobin levels may also be congenital (albeit rarely in Europe). They may also be observed in other, non-hemolytic diseases, e.g. in liver diseases and in malabsorption syndrome. Since the LDH concentration in the erythrocytes is about 360 times higher than in the plasma, with hemolytic processes there is a rise in LDH. The LDH increase stands in direct relationship to the erythrocyte destruction. A particularly large rise in LDH can be observed in hemolytic crises. Hemolytic anemia caused by a circulatory trauma is characterized by the occurrence of burr and helmet cells. The most important causes of hemolytic anemia are listed in Table 40.

Table 40: Mechanically induced forms of hemolytic anemia

Microangiopathies
- Splenomegaly
- Hemolytic uremic syndrome (HUS)
- Thrombotic thrombocytopenic purpura (TTP)
- Cirrhosis of the liver
- Eclampsia
Prosthetic heart valves
Extracorporeal pump systems
- Hemodialysis
- Hemofiltration
- Extracorporeal oxygenation

Corpuscular Anemias

The most important of the enzyme defects is glucose-6-phosphate dehydrogenase deficiency with all its genetically fixed variants, of which favism is now clinically the best known form.

The hemoglobinopathy that has attained most importance is sickle cell anemia in all its variants; Met-hemoglobin (met-Hb) is also worthy of mention as the cause of familiar cyanosis. The hemoglobinopathies also include all variants of thalassemia, a disorder which is gaining importance with the increasing mobility of the world's population. These hemoglobinopathies generally present a variable morphologic picture with target cells. A clear diagnosis can be made only by hemoglobin electrophoresis or by high-pressure liquid chromatography (HPLC).

Erythropoietin Therapy of Other Diseases

Erythropoietin is used successfully in patients with disturbances of iron utilization and distribution, chronic diseases and to promote erythropoiesis in individuals donating blood for their own use in planned orthopedic surgery.

EPO is now produced using recombinant genetic engineering techniques. When expressed in mammalian cells, EPO receives the necessary high portion of carbohydrates. The half-life of intravenously administered EPO is about 5 hours [61].

A very successful therapy with erythropoietin is used with anemic AIDS patients. In patients with hemoblastoses and malignancies on chemotherapy, the suppression of erythropoiesis – which is often a result of intensive chemotherapy – can be overcome with erythropoietin therapy.

A new therapeutic strategy using EPO has been used successfully in treating anemic newborns. Due to the relative hypoxia during intrauterine growth, newborns have a polycythemia. In adapting to the environmental conditions, erythropoiesis is slowed greatly after birth. The reduced erythropoiesis leads to physiologic anemia in newborns after 8–12 weeks. After that, the level of erythropoietin rises once more, and erythropoiesis reaches a normal level. Symptoms of anemia are rarely observed in mature newborns, although aggravating factors occur with premature infants. The number of erythrocytes is lower at birth than in mature newborns, and their erythrocyte life span is shorter. Premature infants therefore often tend to develop anemias.

Approximately 50% of all premature infants have a Hb concentration less than 9 g/dL. This development of anemia can be bridged by the administration of erythropoietin, and it can replace the transfusion therapy used in the past. Additional iron replacement is recommended.

Increasingly, autologous blood donations are being set aside by patients before they undergo a planned surgical procedure in order to avoid the risk of contracting HIV or hepatitis if they should require a blood transfusion. The risk of contracting an infection from a homologous conserved blood donation is about $1:10^6$ for an HIV infection, 1:50,000 for a hepatitis B infection, and 1:5000 for a hepatitis C infection.

The indications for replacement therapy with erythropoietin are increasing. The effectiveness of the therapy must be monitored at all times, however, in order to determine the response rate and to control the therapy.

Clinical Aspects

Methods of Determination

The methods used for determination of plasma proteins and hematological parameters are described here only in principle; the listed references allow the reader to obtain further and more detailed information. The recommended reference intervals apply only to the methods described in the respective references.

The development of new methods, the improvement of existing methods, high quality standards as well as increasing national and international standardization have resulted in an increase in the clinical sensitivity and specificity of clinical laboratory diagnostic investigations. The current international standard is mentioned whenever possible.

Parameters in Serum/Plasma

In addition to blood count and hematocrit, the diagnostics of disturbances in iron metabolism is based on the investigation of a number of parameters in serum and plasma:

- Iron
- Hemoglobin (Hb)
- Total iron-binding capacity (TIBC)
- Latent iron-binding capacity (LIBC)
- Ferritin
- Transferrin (Tf)
- Transferrin saturation (TfS)
- Soluble transferrin receptor (sTfR)
- Haptoglobin (Hp)
- Ceruloplasmin (Cp)
- Folic acid
- Vitamin B_{12}
- Erythropoietin (EPO)
- Homocysteine
- Methylmalonic acid
- Holotranscobalamin

Iron

In addition to the colorimetric methods, which are by far the most commonly used, atomic absorption spectrophotometry (AAS) and potentiostatic coulometry are also available as special techniques. More than 95% of all iron determinations in clinical laboratories are performed colorimetrically using routine analyzers.

All the colorimetric methods developed for the determination of iron have the following steps in common:

- Liberation of the Fe^{3+} ions from the transferrin complex by acids or tensides.
- Reduction of Fe^{3+} ions to Fe^{2+} ions by ascorbate, thioglycolate, or hydroxylamine.
- Reaction of the Fe^{2+} ions to form a colored complex

The complexing agents used nowadays are bathophenanthroline and FerroZine® (Hach Chemical Co., Ames, Iowa/USA). FerroZine® has a higher extinction coefficient than bathophenanthroline and its solubility is also better.

Reference methods for the determination of serum/plasma iron have been proposed by the International Committee for Standardization in Hematology (ICSH) [75] and more recently by the Center of Disease Control (CDC) [144].

The method recommended in 1972 by the ICSH uses 2 mol/L hydrochloric acid for the liberation and thioglycolic acid for the reduction of the Fe^{3+} ions. The complexing agent in the ICSH reagent is bathophenanthroline-disulfonate.

The CDC proposal is a method with sample deproteinization by trichloroacetic acid, and with reduction by ascorbic acid. The complexing agent is FerroZine®.

The various methods available for the determination of iron on routine clinical chemistry analyzers generally do not involve a precipitation step.

The serum iron level shows a distinct circadian rhythm. There is also a considerable day-to-day variation. In serum, iron is bound to proteins. The collection of blood samples must therefore be standardized with respect to time, body position, and venous occlusion.

Iron is one of the trace elements, with a concentration in the serum similar to those of copper and zinc. Contamination must therefore be avoided during the collection and preparation of samples.

Serum and heparinized plasma are suitable for use as samples. EDTA plasma cannot be used. Hemolysis interferes. No detectable change in the iron concentration is found upon storage of serum for several weeks at +4 °C.

Reference Range

Reference range for serum/plasma iron in healthy subjects [67]:

Women	37–145 µg/dL	6.6–26 µmol/L
Men	59–158 µg/dL	11–28 µmol/L

Note

Considerable differenct iron reference ranges are given in the literature. There are various reasons for this:

- The reference range does not show a normal distribution.
- Iron concentrations found for men are about 15–20% higher than those for women.
- A significant fraction of the "normal population" may suffer from latent iron deficiency, depending on the dietary habits.
- Intra-individual iron concentrations in serum/plasma show considerable day-to-day fluctuations (Fig. 43).

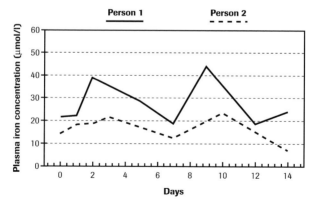

Fig. 43: Day-to-day fluctuations of the plasma iron concentration

Iron Saturation (Total Iron-Binding Capacity and Latent Iron-Binding Capacity)

These methods have now been largely replaced by the determination of transferrin and of the transferrin saturation.

The Total Iron-Binding Capacity (TIBC) is the quantity of iron that can be bound by transferrin in a specified volume of serum.

The Latent Iron-Binding Capacity (LIBC) is the result obtained when the quantity of iron actually present is subtracted from the TIBC. The following relation exists:

$$TIBC = LIBC + Plasma \ Iron$$

The TIBC is measured in the routine laboratory according to Ramsay, and is performed in parallel with the determination of iron: An excess of Fe^{3+} ions is added to the serum to saturate the transferrin. The unbound Fe^{3+} ions are then precipitated with basic magnesium carbonate. After centrifugation, the iron in the clear supernatant is measured.

Iron-Binding Proteins

All methods for the determination of plasma proteins such as ferritin and transferrin are based on the reaction between an antigen and an antibody. This reaction leads to the formation of an immune complex of antigen.

The initially formed antigen-antibody complex cannot be observed directly if the antigen concentration is very low. In this case either the antigen or the antibody must be labeled in order to make a measurement possible. The label may be, e.g. an enzyme, a radioactive isotope, a luminescence-producing substance, or a fluorescent dye. These indirect methods are particularly suitable for the determination of very low antigen concentrations, as in the case of ferritin. The indirect methods require an extra step to remove unbound antibody or antigen usually from a solid phase reagent (heterogeneous immunoassay).

With higher antigen concentrations, the initial reaction between the antigen and the antibody may be followed by agglutination or precipitation as a secondary reaction. The results can then be measured directly, and are often visible. These direct methods are particularly suitable for

Laboratory

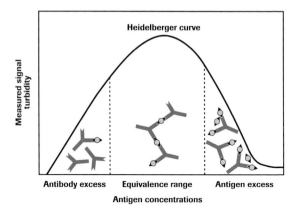

Fig. 44: Heidelberger-Kendall curve

the determination of higher antigen concentrations as e.g., in the case of transferrin.

In all direct immunoassays the quantitative determination is based on the Heidelberger-Kendall curve [66], which describes the relationship between the antigen concentration and the quantity of precipitate for a constant quantity of antibody. The quantity of precipitate is measured photometrically or nephelometrically (Fig. 44).

As can be seen from the course of the Heidelberger curve (Fig. 44), two different antigen concentrations can give the same measurement signal. This can lead to incorrect results. Quantitative immunoassays must therefore be performed below the equivalence point. The conventional method of deciding whether a signal lies on the ascending (antibody excess) or descending (antigen excess) part of the Heidelberger curve is to repeat the determination with a higher dilution of the sample. Another possibility is to add antigen or antiserum to the reaction mixture. Modern automated analyzers can virtually eliminate this source of error by means of check functions (characterization and automatic redilution of the sample). Most manufacturers of immunochemical reagents declare the concentration range in which no antigen excess problem arises, i.e., no high-dose hook effect is found.

To enhance the sensitivity, antibodies coated to microparticles are used in the direct immunoassays (particle- or latex-enhanced immunoassays).

To combine high analytical sensitivity with wide dynamic measuring range a mixture of larger particles coated with a high-reactivity antibody and smaller particles coated with a low-reactivity antibody are used.

The high-reactivity antibody reacts very quickly with the antigen leading to a strong measuring signal at very low analyte concentrations. This reaction is dominating at low analyte concentration and provides the desired high analytical sensitivity. The low-affinity antibody provides less analytical sensitivity but enables a high upper measuring limit.

The direct, homogeneous methods do not require separation steps and all components of the assay are present during the measurement. Compared to indirect immunoassays the incubation times are short.

Two different measuring principles are applied:

Turbidimetry: A light beam passing through the reaction mixture is weakend by its turbidity caused by antigen/antibody aggregates, which can be measured with a photometer. The consolidated measurement of serum proteins, drugs, and conventional clinical chemical parameters on one instrument is possible.

Nephelometry: A light beam passing through the reaction mixture is scattered by the antigen-antibody aggregates. The intensity of the scattered light is proportional to the amount of antigen-antibody aggregates. The measurement of scattered light intensity allows the quantification of the analyte using a calibration curve.

Ferritin

The ferritin that can be detected in the blood is in equilibrium with the body's storage iron, and can thus serve as an index of the size of the iron stores.

Ferritin does not represent a uniform molecular entity. It occurs in different tissues as various isoferritins. These isoferritins are constructed from two subunits, the H-(heavy)-type subunit and the L-(light)-type subunit (Fig. 45).

For the clinical evaluation of the body's iron stores by the determination of ferritin, the ferritin antibodies must possess specificity for the basic L-rich isoferritins from iron storage tissues (marrow, liver, and spleen), whereas their reactivity with acidic H-rich isoferritins (e.g., from cardiac muscle) should be as low as possible.

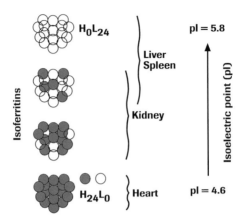

Fig. 45: Organ-specific isoferritins

Latex-enhanced immunoassay tests are particularly suitable for the detection of the very low plasma ferritin concentration ($0.2–7 \times 10^{-12}$ mol/L). But heterogenous immunoassays are also used for the determination of ferritin.

International efforts toward a uniform standardization of ferritin are being coordinated by the WHO (World Health Organization), the ICSH (International Committee of Standardization in Hematology), the IFCC (International Federation of Clinical Chemistry), and the IUIS (Standardization Committee of the International Union of Immunological Societies).

The prerequisite for uniform standardization of ferritin assays is a defined ferritin preparation with a high content of basic isoferritins. Such a ferritin standard (human liver ferritin) is available from the ICHS (Expert Panel of Iron) since 1984. Since 1997 the WHO 3rd International Standard for Ferritin, recombinant (94/572) is available [141].

Ferritin, like transferrin, but unlike iron, shows no appreciable circadian rhythm. In view of the effect of an upright body position on high molecular weight blood components, the blood collection conditions must be standardized with regard to body position and venous occlusion.

Preferably the same sample should be used for the ferritin determinations as for the iron, transferrin, and soluble transferrin receptor (sTfR).

Reference Range

The ferritin concentrations in serum/plasma are dependent on age and sex (Fig. 46), and on the standardization of the specific assay. This limits the interlaboratory comparability of ferritin test results.

Using an electroluminescence immunoassay and a turbidimetric immunoassay with uniform standardization the following reference ranges were found in healthy adults [67]:

Females	15–150 µg/L
Males	30–400 µg/L

Note

- Babies initially have full iron stores, which are used up within a few weeks.

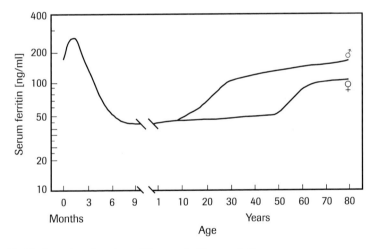

Fig. 46: Age and sex dependence of the serum ferritin concentration

Transferrin

Half of the body's transferrin (Tf) is contained in the serum/plasma, while the other half is extravascular. The protein is able to transport two trivalent iron ions per molecule. 30–40% of this maximum binding capacity is utilized under physiologic conditions.

Transferrin is not a uniform molecule. It represents a group of various isotransferrins. Approximately 20 human isotransferrins are known. They all have the same iron-binding capacity and similar immunologic characteristics. Therefore distinguishing between the various isoforms has no practical value for the assessment of iron metabolism. Since the technical requirements for the determination of transferrin in the routine laboratory are relatively simple, the determination of transferrin in serum/plasma has largely displaced the determination of the TIBC (total iron-binding capacity) and of the LIBC (latent iron-binding capacity). The relationship between transferrin and total iron-binding capacity (TIBC) is illustrated in Table 41.

Table 41: Relationship between transferrin and TIBC

Relation between transferrin and TIBC	Reference ranges
Tsf [µmol/L] × 2 ≈ TIBC [µmol/L]	Tsf: 16–45 µmol/L TIBC, W: 49–89 µmol/L TIBC, M: 52–77 µmol/L
$\text{Tsf [mg/dL]} \times \dfrac{2 \times 56}{79{,}570} \approx \text{TIBC [µg/dL]}$	Tsf: 130–160 mg/L TIBC, W: 274–497 mg/L TIBC, M: 291–430 mg/L

*1 mol of transferrin binds 2 atoms of iron, atomic weight of iron: 56 D, molecular weight of apo-transferrin: 79,570 D [64].

Methods

Because of its relatively high concentration in serum/plasma, direct immunologic precipitation methods (nephelometric and turbidimetric) are suitable for transferrin determination in these specimens.

Transferrin, like ferritin, but unlike iron, shows no pronounced circadian rhythm. In view of the effect of an upright body position on high molecular weight blood components, the blood collection conditions for transferrin determinations must again be standardized with regard to body position and vein constriction. Preferably the same sample should be used for the transferrin determination as for iron and ferritin.

Reference Range

No major dependence on age or sex was found [67].

Adults	130–360 mg/dL (16–45 μmol/L)

Note

Total Iron-Binding Capacity (TIBC) of 1 g transferrin is 1.41 mg iron.

Transferrin Saturation

Transferrin saturation (TfS) is defined as the ratio of the serum/plasma iron concentration to the serum/plasma transferrin concentration (multiplied by a correction factor). It is a dimensionless quantity, so that unlike iron, it is independent of the patient's state of hydration:

$$\text{Transferrin saturation [\%]:} \frac{\text{Iron [μmol/L]} \times 100}{\text{Transferrin [μmol/L]}}$$

or:

$$\frac{\text{Iron [μg/dL]} \times 100 \times 56}{\text{Transferrin [μg/dL]} \times 79{,}570}$$

56: atomic weight of iron
79,570: atomic weight of apotransferrin

Reference Range [67]

Transferrin saturation in healthy individuals	16–45%
Decreased transferrin saturation in iron deficiency or disturbances of iron distribution	<15%
Elevated transferrin saturation in iron overload	>50%

Note

Transferrin saturation of 50% is reached, when 1 g transferrin contains 0.705 mg iron. Transferrin saturation of 10% expresses that 1 g transferrin is loadeded with 0.141 mg iron.

Laboratory

Laboratory

Soluble Transferrin Receptor

The transferrin receptor (sTfR) is a transmembrane dimeric glycoprotein of many cells of the body. It is made of two identical subunits which are connected via disulfide bonds. Its molecular weight is 190,000 D. Its function is to bind iron-loaded transferrin and to transport it into the cell.

The transferrin receptor is found in a soluble form in serum/plasma. This soluble transferrin receptor (sTfR) is a monomer of approximately 85,000 D. It is generated by proteolytic cleavage between Arg-100 and Leu-101 of the transferrin receptor monomers [38, 73].

Particle-enhanced immunonephelometric and turbidimetric tests are currently the methods most frequently used for routine determinations of sTfR. A sTfR reference standard is not yet available. To calibrate the assays, human serum-based preparations of intact TfR, the complex of TfR with transferrin or mixtures are used. Therefore, the interassay comparability of sTfR results is limited.

Reference ranges [83]

| Females (premenopausal) | 1.9–4.4 mg/L |
| Males | 2.2–5.0 mg/L |

There is a good direct proportional relationship between the serum/plasma concentration of sTfR and
- the amount of TfR on the erythrocytes
- the mass of erythropoietic cells.

The concentration of sTfR is therefore raised in the presence of increased expression of TfR, as is the case with active iron deficiency, and in hyper-proliferative erythropoiesis. These states can be differentiated by performing additional determinations of ferritin and reticulocyte count.

Haptoglobin

The biosynthesis of haptoglobin occurs not only in the liver, but also in adipose tissue and in lung. It is a glycoprotein structurally related to the immunoglobulins, and is made up of 2 (α) light chains with a molecular weight of 9000 D and two heavier (β) chains (molecular weight: 16,000 D). Three phenotypes with different molecular weights are known: Hp1–1, Hp2–1 and Hp2–2. Hp1–1 has a molecular weight of 100,000 D. Hp2–1 and Hp2–2 are high-molecular-weight polymers with a molecular weight ranging from 200,000 to 400,000 D. The site of haptoglobin synthesis is the liver.

Haptoglobin is an acute-phase protein. One of its functions is to bind free hemoglobin in the blood resulting from hemolysis thus preventing iron loss and renal damage. A stable 1:1 haptoglobin-hemoglobin (Hp-Hb) complex is formed which is eliminated from the circulation with a half-life of 8 min by receptor-mediated uptake into the cells of the RES. The hemoglobin is then intracellularly degraded, the iron contained in the heme is liberated and recirculated to the metabolism. The haptoglobin released is returned to the serum with a half-life of about 3 days.

Since with pathologically increased hemolysis the production of haptoglobin does not keep pace with its consumption, a decrease in the concentration of free haptoglobin in serum/plasma thus can serve as an indicator of intravascular hemolysis.

In the presence of massive hemolysis – when no haptoglobin concentration is detectable – hemopexin (Hpx) should be measured.

Methods

Because of the relatively high haptoglobin concentration in the serum, immunonephelometric and turbidimetric tests are currently the methods most frequently used for routine determinations.

Reference Range

Like ferritin and transferrin, haptoglobin shows no appreciable circadian rhythm. There are no major differences based on age or sex [67].

Adults	0.30–2.00 g/L

Note

- Neonates have no measurable haptoglobin levels in the first 3 months; the reference range for adults applies from the 4th month of life.

- Haptoglobin shows a genetic polymorphism which leads to three phenotypes differing in molecular weight: Hp 1-1 (Africa, South, and Central America), Hp 2-1 (Asia) and Hp 2-2 (Central Europe) [67] (Table 42).

Table 42: Dependence of haptoglobin reference range on phenotype and gender

Phenotype	Gender	Reference range [g/L]
Hp1–1	w	0.91–1.60
	m	0.87–1.42
Hp2–1	w	0.82–1.24
	m	0.74–1.24
Hp2–2	w	0.58–0.99
	m	0.52–1.01

Ceruloplasmin

Ceruloplasmin (Cp) is also known as ferroxidase or iron(II): oxygen oxidoreductase. It is an α-glycoprotein with a molecular mass of 132 kDa and is synthesized mostly in the liver. Cp has 8 binding sites for Cu^{2+} ions and is the major copper-carrying protein in the blood. Additionally, it has a copper-dependent catalytical function in the intracellular oxidation of Fe^{2+} into Fe^{3+}, which is necessary for the release of iron ions from the cells and the binding to transferrin. Therefore, it is assisting in the transport of iron in the plasma (transferrin can carry only iron in the Fe^{3+} state).

This is exemplified by the very rare hereditary aceruloplasminemia where the lack of iron oxidation prevents binding of iron to transferrin and thereby leads to intracellular trapping of iron ions and consequently to the development of an iron overload which resembles hereditary hemochromatosis. In contrast to hemochromatosis the central nervous system is also affected. Due to the impaired transferrin binding, however, iron concentrations and transferrin saturation in plasma are low in these cases whereas the ferritin concentration is high, reflecting impaired iron distribution and release. Therefore, in this disease disturbance of iron distribution occurs in addition to the iron overload [78].

Laboratory

Methods

In the routine clinical chemistry laboratory immunoturbidimetric or immunonephelometric methods are used for the determination of Cp.

Reference Range

There are no major differences based on age or sex [67].

Adults	15–60 mg/dL (0.15–0.6 g/L)

Vitamin B₁₂

Vitamin B_{12} has a molecular weight of 1355 daltons and, as cyanocobalamin, belongs to a group of biologically active substances which have as common structural element a porphyrin ring with cobalt(III) as the central ion.

The vitamin B_{12} taken up with food or synthesized by intestinal bacteria ("extrinsic factor") forms a complex with the "intrinsic factor", a glycoprotein secreted by the gastric mucosa. Formation of this complex serves to protect the vitamin from degradation in the intestine and facilitates its receptor-dependent absorption by the mucosa of the small intestine. After dissociation of the vitamin B_{12} – "intrinsic factor" complex the vitamin can be transported to the liver, where it is stored. In the cells, the vitamin is present mainly as 5′-deoxyadenosylcobalamin, whereas methylcobalamin predominates in the plasma. The main transport protein for vitamin B_{12} in plasma is transcobalamin II (TC-II).

Methods

A microbiologic assay is recommended by the NCCLS as reference method for the research laboratory. The concentration of vitamin B_{12} is determined as measured in relation to its biologic activity to promote the growth of *Euglena gracilis* or *Lactobacillus leichmannii*. However, this method is not suitable for wider use because of the apparatus required and the cumbersome technique.

Before the determination is performed, vitamin B_{12} is released from the endogenous binding proteins by heating or by pretreatment in an alkaline solution.

Radioassays were first reported for vitamin B_{12} in 1961 [12]. They utilized ^{57}Co-cyanocobalamin-labeled tracers and intrinsic factor for binding vitamin B_{12}. The presence of endogenous serum-binding proteins for cyanocobalamin (transcobalamins including R protein) and of immunoglobulins directed against intrinsic factor require that specimens are either boiled or treated at an alkaline pH to release the vitamin B_{12}.

In the late 1970s, radioassays using serum-binding proteins or partially purified intrinsic factor measured levels of vitamin B_{12} which exceeded those determined by the microbiologic methods. This was caused by the presence of the R proteins in the assay. R protein specificity is poor compared to that of intrinsic factor and vitamin B_{12} analogs were being measured in addition to vitamin B_{12} itself [153]. Since that time, recommendations have been established for the use of highly purified intrinsic factor throughout the industry.

The various commercial assays differ in their detection system, free versus bound separation techniques, and choice of specimen pretreatment.

Reference Range

There are no major differences based on age or sex [67].

Adults	220–925 pg/mL (162–683 pmol/L)

Note

- The body's vitamin B_{12} pool is approximately 3–7 mg. Given a requirement of 30 µg/d, parental administration of vitamin B_{12} often leads to raised concentrations after a few months.
- In about 20% of pregnant women, the vitamin B_{12} concentration in serum falls to values of <125 pmol/L despite adequate depots.
- Reference ranges for vitamin B_{12} given in the literature may differ considerably. This is undoubtedly due to the differences in methodologies.

Holotrancobalamin

About 70–90% of vitamin B_{12} in serum is bound to haptocorrin (HC). This transport form of vitamin B_{12} (HoloHC) can be taken up only by liver cells. The remaining 10–30% of vitamin B_{12} is bound to transcobalamin II (HoloTC). HoloTC is taken up by the peripheral cells via a receptor-mediated process and vitamin B_{12} is thus made available for the cellular metabolism. Then measurement of HoloHC is of special importance since it is the only marker which is indicative for early stages of vitamin B_{12} deficiency.

Method
A microparticle enzyme immunoassay is available for holotranscobalamin determination.

Reference Range [120]

Women	19–45 yr	34–141 pmol/L
	46–69 yr	48–174 pmol/L
Men	18–45 yr	46–152 pmol/L
	46–68 yr	41–176 pmol/L

Note
To confirm intracellular vitamin B_{12} deficiency, the determination of methylmalonic acid (MMA) may be performed. With intracellular vitamin B_{12} deficiency MMA, like homocysteine, accumulates in the cells leading to increased MMA release into the circulation. The reference range of serum MMA is 9–32 ng/mL; increased values are found with intracellular vitamin B_{12} deficiency.

Folic Acid

Folic acid is a pteridine derivative and is present as a conjugate with several glutaminic acid molecules. After the ingestion it is initially hydrolyzed enzymatically to pteroylmonoglutaminic acid (PGA) in the mucosal epithelium of the small intestine. Reduction and methylation then take place in the intestinal wall; the resultant N-5-methyltetrahydrofolic acid (MTHFA) is released into the bloodstream. Tetrahydrofolic acid (THFA) is formed from MTHFA. Vitamin B_{12} is required for this conversion. THFA is involved in numerous reactions as an acceptor and donor of single carbon groups, especially in the synthesis of purines, pyrimidines, glycine, and methionine.

Methods

The microbiologic assay recommended as reference method is not suited for routine use.

A major advance in methods was achieved in 1973 with the introduction of the radioimmunologic competitive protein-binding test. The determination is based on the competitive binding of [125]J-labeled N-5-methyltetrahydrofolic acid (MTHFA) of the sample to the milk-binding protein (3-lactoglobulin). Before the determination is performed, MTHFA is released from the endogenous binding proteins by boiling or by pretreatment in an alkaline solution. The false normal results observed in individual cases which, compared with the microbiologic reference method, failed to reveal a folic acid deficiency, can be corrected using chromatographically highly purified 3-lactoglobulin free from non-specific binding proteins.

The majority of assays currently in routine use utilize non-radioactive tracers, natural binding proteins (milk-binding protein and folate-binding protein), and "non-boil" sample pretreatment. They differ mainly in their free versus bound separation techniques and pretreatment procedures.

Since more than 95% of folate occurs in the red blood cells, the folate concentration in erythrocytes more truly reflects the overall folate concentration in the tissue. Therefore, it is recommended to perform folate determinations not only in serum/plasma but also in erythrocytes (RBC folate). In these assays whole blood treated with anticoagulants (heparin or EDTA) is diluted and preincubated with a solution containing a reducing agent prior to the assay.

Reference Ranges [67]

Folate, serum	3.8 – 16.0 ng/mL	8.6 – 36.3 nmol/L
Folate, red blood cells	416 – 1367 ng/mL	597 – 3103 nmol/L

Note

Because of the close connection between vitamin B_{12} and folic acid in the metabolism and the difficulty of hematologic and clinical differentiation between the two vitamin deficiency states, it is advisable to determine both parameters simultaneously in patients with the relevant vitamin deficiency symptoms.

- Given a requirement of approximately 200 µg/d and a total content in the body of about 5–10 mg, parental administration of folic acid (e.g., in absorption tests) often leads to raised concentrations of folic acid after a few weeks.
- Some of the reference ranges for folic acid given in the literature differ considerably. This is undoubtedly due to the differences in methodologies used in the past.
- Findings of Brouwer [27] suggest that the reference ranges for folic acid should be increased.

Homocysteine

Homocysteine is a sulfur-containing intermediary product in methionine metabolism. As a consequence of the biochemical reactions in which homocysteine is involved, deficiencies of folic acid, vitamin B_6 (pyridoxine), or vitamin B_{12} (cyanocobalamin) can lead to increased homocysteine levels. A high serum homocysteine level is a marker for cardiovascular disease.

Methods
Chromatographic, enzymatic, and immunoassays are available to measure homocysteine. The immunoassays include fluorescent immunoassay, chemiluminescent immunoassay, and microtiter plate platforms. Chromatographic based methods include HPLC with fluorescent or electrochemical detection, gas chromatography, and liquid chromatography with single or tandem mass spectrometry. In the enzymatic methods the amount of NADH converted to NAD is measured, which is indirectly proportional to the concentration of homocysteine in the sample. One of these enzymatic methods is based on an enzyme cycling principle that assesses a co-substrate conversion product instead of assessing the co-substrate or the conversion products of homocysteine. By these means the detection signal is significantly amplified.

Laboratory

Reference Ranges [67]

Females	<30 yr	0.8–1.9 mg/L	6–14 μmol/L
	30–59 yr	0.7–1.8 mg/L	5–13 μmol/L
	>60 yr	0.9–1.9 mg/L	7–14 μmol/L
Males	<30 yr	0.8–1.9 mg/L	6–14 μmol/L
	30–59 yr	0.8–2.2 mg/L	6–16 μmol/L
	>60–84 yr	0.8–2.3 mg/L	6–17 μmol/L
	>85 yr	2.0–4.0 mg/L	15–30 μmol/L

Erythropoietin

The focus of erythropoietin determination in clinical diagnostics lies in the differential diagnosis of erythrocytosis. Other indications are suspicion of renal anemia and determination of the starting value before initiating treatment of anemia with rhu-EPO. Interpretation of the measured EPO concentration is only possible in conjunction with hemoglobin or hematocrit levels (Fig. 47). Both a decrease and an increase in the production of EPO are of diagnostic significance.

EPO deficiency causes normocytic normochromic anemia. The most common cause is chronic renal failure because in adults EPO is almost exclusively synthesized in the kidney.

Table 43: Properties of erythropoietin

Molecular properties	• EPO is an acidic glycoprotein.
	• The non-processed protein consists of 193 amino acids. To form the "mature" EPO polypeptide, a 27-amino acid-fragment is split from the N-terminus, and a single arginine group is split from the C-terminus.
	• The processed protein consists of 165 amino acids.
	• EPO contains two disulfide bonds, at least one of which is important for the biologic activity of the hormone.
	• The individual polypeptide chain is responsible for stimulating the target cells.
	• The four carbohydrate side chains determine the stability and pharmacokinetic properties of the molecule (in particular the rate at which EPO is eliminated from the circulation).
Molecular weight	• Depending on carbohydrate side chains, the molecular weight is between 30,000 and 34,000 D.

Laboratory

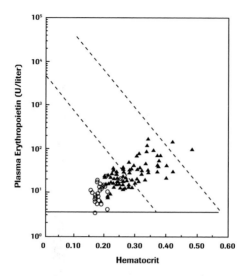

Fig. 47: Plasma erythropoietin levels in 120 patients receiving dialysis in relation to hematocrit. From [48]

○ patients without kidneys, ▲ patients with kidneys, ---- 95% confidence interval for 175 normal blood donors and patients with anemia, ——— lower detection limit of test.

Reference Range

There are no major differences related to age or gender [67].

Adults	5–25 IU/L

Blood Count

The complete blood cell count of the small (red) and large (red and white) blood count is performed today using modern, fully automated hematology analyzers. The wide variety of hematology systems offered on the market today differ according to:

- Level of automation. Systems range from semi-automated, automated, and fully-automated analyzers with different methods of sample pretreatment and sample delivery
- Standardization and quality assurance
- Number of analytical parameters

Laboratory

Whole blood anticoagulated with EDTA is used as the sample. The following parameters are determined or calculated:

- Hemoglobin (Hb)
- Hematocrit (HCT)
- Red blood cell (RBC) count
- Erythrocyte indices
  - Mean cell volume (MCV) of the red cells
  - Mean cell hemoglobin (MCH) content of red cells
  - Mean cell hemoglobin concentration (MCHC) of red cells
  - Red cell distribution width (RDW)
- Reticulocyte count
  - Mean cell volume reticulocytes (MCVr)
  - Mean cell hemoglobin concentration reticulocytes (CHCMr)
- Hemoglobin content reticulocyte (CHr). CHr is the product of $MCVr \times CHCMr = CHr$

Table 44: Parameters determined in routine hematology

Parameter	Complete blood count	Differential blood count
Number and type of blood cells	WBC RBC PLC	*3-Part differential* Lymphocytes Monocytes Granulocytes
		5-Part differential Lymphocytes Monocytes Neutrophils Basophils Eosinophils
Hb concentration	Hb	
(Red blood) cell vol. as % of total blood volume	Htc or PCV	
Red blood cell indices to define size and Hb content of RBCs (calculated using Hb, RBC, and Hct)	MCV MCH MCHC	

Hb, hemoglobin; Htc, hematocrit; MCH, mean cell Hb; MCHC, mean cell Hb concentration; MCV, mean cell volume; PLC, platelet count, PCV, packed cell volume.

- White blood cell (WBC) count
- Differentiated count leukocytes (DCL, number of lymphocytes, mono-cytes, neutrophils, basophils and eosinophils)
- Platelet (PLT) count
- Mean platelet volume (MPV).

The so-called small blood count comprises the parameters RBC, Hb, HCT, MCV, MCH, MCHC, WBC, and PLT).

Automated Cell Counting

Today, automated hematology systems, either impedance-based or based on optical principles, are routinely used in many hematologic laboratories.

Flow Cytometry

The principles of light scattering, light excitation, and light emission of fluorochrome molecules to generate specific multi-parameter data from particles e.g., nuclei) and cells contained in blood and other body fluids are applied in flow cytometry [133].

The sample is injected into the center of a sheath flow. The cells or particles are hydro-dynamically focused before intercepting an optimal-ly focused laser beam. The combined flow is reduced in diameter, forc-ing the cells into the center of the stream. Thus the laser beam is intercepted by one cell at a time.

Each suspended particle passing through the laser beam scatters the light in some way, and fluorescent chemicals found in the particle or attached to the particle may be excited into emitting light at a lower frequency than the light source. This combination of scattered and fluo-rescent light is picked up by detectors, and by analyzing fluctuations in brightness at each detector (one for each fluorescent emission peak) it is then possible to derive various types of information about the physical and chemical structures of each individual cell or particle.

The electrical pulses originating from light detected by the photo-multiplier tubes of the flow cytometer are processed by a series of linear

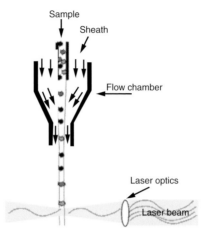

Fig. 48: Principles of flow cytometry

and log amplifiers. Logarithmic amplification is most often used to measure fluorescence in cells. This type of amplification expands the scale for weak signals and compresses the scale for "strong" or specific fluorescence signals.

The scattered light is evaluated at different angles thus defining different characteristics of the cells or particles involved. The scatter characteristics strongly depend on the wavelength of the light and the

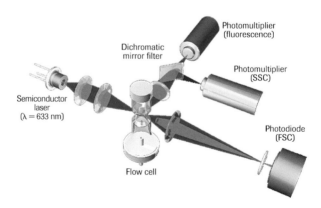

Fig. 49: Schematic illustration of a flow cytometer

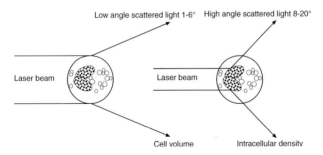

Fig. 50: Principle of flow cytometric cellular volume and intracellular density measurements

particle size. For example, low-angle scattered light reflects cell size, and right angle (orthogonal or side scatter) reflects intracellular structure.

Depending on the application or staining technique used, either protein-fluorochrome conjugates such as fluorescent-labeled antibodies or affinity-bound dyes, e.g., thiazole orange, for reticulocyte RNA staining, is available.

For reticulocyte analysis the cells are labelled with a fluorescent dye which specifically stains the nucleic acids of the reticulate cells. Since the nucleic acid content of the reticulocytes decreases during the maturation process until they turn into mature erythrocytes the fluorescence emitted by them can be used for reticulocyte differentiation.

During the cell count in the flow cytometer, the fluorescence intensity as well as the intensity of the forward scatter of every single stained cell is measured. Thus, information is obtained about the nucleic acid content and size of every cell. The different degrees of maturation of the reticulocytes correspond to the intensity of the emitted light. The fractions HFR (high fluorescence intensity of reticulocytes), MFR (mean fluorescence intensity of reticulocytes) and LRF (low fluorescence intensity of reticulocytes) are determined. Moreover, the population of very early reticulocytes – the immature reticulocyte fraction (IRF) – is analyzed.

The IRF value and the degrees of maturity are proven parameters for assessing the hematopoietic activity of the bone marrow. This information can be used to assess the status of the red cell line.

Modern flow cytometers are able to analyze several thousand particles or cells every second, offering "high-throughput" (for a large num-

Laboratory

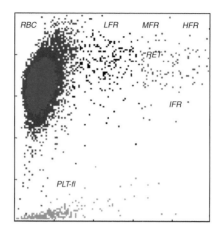

Fig. 51: Flow cytometer scattergram, classification of reticulocytes (degree of maturity)

RBC: mature erythrocytes; RET: reticulocytes; HFR: high fluoresence intensity of reticulocytes; MFR: mean fluoresence intensity of reticulocytes; LFR: low fluoresence intensity of reticulocytes; IRF: immature reticulocyte fraction; PLT-fl: fluorescence thrombocytes

ber of cells) automated quantification of set parameters. Typically, 5–6 parameters are measured simultaneously, e.g., cell size, intracellular density, and fluorescences of various colors. Modern instruments usually have multiple lasers and fluorescence detectors, allowing for multiple antibody labeling, and more precise identification of a target particle or cell population.

Impedance-Based Cell Counters

EDTA blood is diluted with a defined volume of electrolyte solution and placed in a transducer chamber which is connected with a further electrolyte solution via a small orifice (50–100 mm). A constant electric current is applied between electrodes on either side of the orifice. The cell suspension is drawn through the measuring orifice by means of a vacuum. When a cell passes through the orifice it acts as non-conducter and the resistance increases. Using Ohm's law, a pulse proportionate to the volume can be derived (Fig. 52). In systems using absolute measure-

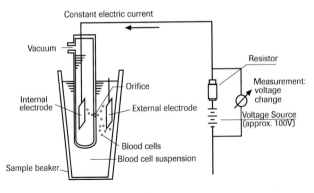

Fig. 52: Impedance-based particle counting instrument. Schematic diagram

ment (number of cells per volume), the counting volume is determined with the help of manometers. Systems using the principle of relative measurement determine the cell count per unit of time. In this case the counting rate must then be converted to the cell count per volume with the help of a calibration solution (Fig. 53).

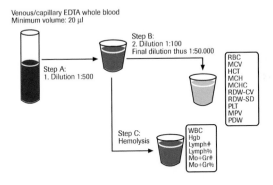

Fig. 53: Sample preparation for a semiautomatic cell counter, blood count panel

RBC: erythrocytes; MCV: mean cellular volume; HCT: hematocrit; MCH: mean corpuscular hemoglobin; MCHC: mean corpuscular hemoglobin concentration; RDW-CV, RDW-SD: coefficient of variation, standard deviation of red cell distribution width; PLT: platelet count; MPV: mean platelet volume; PDW: platelet distribution width; WBC: white blood cell count; HgB: hemoglobin; Lymph#, Lymph%: absolute, % lymphocyte count in WBC; Mo+Gr#, Mo+Gr%: absolute, % monocyte +granulocyte count in WBC

Laboratory

The measuring principle for particle counting illustrated in Fig. 52 permits the counting of red cells, white cells, and platelets. On account of their different concentrations in blood, these cells must be counted in two different dilutions (Fig. 53).

In a first dilution the white cells are counted after the erythrocytes have been lysed by a lysing agent. In a second higher dilution the red cells, and platelets are counted. On account of their different sizes, red cells and platelets can be differentiated from each by pulse thresholds known as discriminators. Many systems use variable thresholds i.e., the ideal discriminators are determined for each sample measured. This prevents parts of a cell population from being cut off and therefore not included in the count.

Hemoglobin

The hemoglobins in the blood comprise a group of hemoglobin derivatives, namely:

- Deoxyhemoglobin (HHb)
- Oxyhemoglobin (O_2Hb)
- Carboxyhemoglobin (COHb)
- Hemiglobin (Hi), or methemoglobin (MetHb)

These hemoglobin derivatives, which are present in cell-bound form, are determined as total hemoglobin (Hb) in whole blood. Free hemoglobin, that is the hemoglobin released from the red blood cells, however, is determined in plasma.

Methods

Photometric measurement of hemoglobin is an integral part of present-day hematology systems. The measurement is performed either with part of the leukocyte dilution, in which case the hemoglobin released by lysis of the red cells is transformed into stable derivatives and measured photometrically, or in a separate dilution with a lysing agent specially designed for hemoglobin determination. The latter procedure has the advantage that the lysing agent used is optimized for hemoglobin measurement. There is therefore no need to take into account the sensitivity of the leukocytes and the dilution ration most appropriate for hemoglobin determination can be used. Therefore, a separate hemoglobin channel with a separate hemoglobin lysing agent is subject to less interference by high leukocyte concentrations than hemoglobin photometry as part of the WBC counting.

For hemoglobin determination the cyanmethemoglobin method can be used. This technique has the disadvantage that the solution contains cyanide and must therefore be disposed of as toxic waste.

In this method, the Fe^{2+} of hemoglobin is oxidized to Fe^{3+} by potassium ferricyanide $[K_3Fe(CN)_6]$ forming hemiglobin (Hi). This reacts with the cyanide ions (CN^-), forming cyanmethemoglobin (HiCN). The absorbance of HiCN is measured at 540 nm. The hemiglobincyanide method is the reference method.

Reference Range [67]

Women	12.3–15.3 g/dL	(7.6–9.5 mmol/L)
Men	14.0–17.5 g/dL	(8.7–10.9 mmol/L)

Hematocrit

The hematocrit (Hct), or packed cell volume (PCV), is the ratio of the volume of red cells to the volume of whole blood in a sample of venous or capillary blood. The ratio is measured after appropriate centrifugation. In laboratory practice the hematocrit is usually expressed as a percentage:

$$\text{Hct (\%)}= \frac{\text{Volume}_{\text{Erythrocytes}}}{\text{Volume}_{\text{Whole blood}}} \times 100$$

The hematocrit is a further important parameter in laboratory hematology. This value is also determined automatically by many hematology systems today. Figure 54 shows a schematic comparison of pulse height summation, the method used by many hematology systems, and the centrifugal hematocrit. The cells which pass through the measuring orifice generate pulses which are proportionate to their volume. The hematocrit is obtained by summation of the individual pulses which are between an upper and lower discriminator. The result is multiplied by a constant factor which takes into account the dilution ratio. The

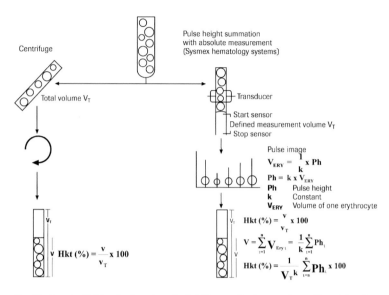

Fig. 54: Hematocrit determination using pulse height summation in comparison with centrifugation

hematocrit represents the percentage by volume of erythrocytes to the total volume of the blood sample. The results of the hematology analyzers are standardized against the microhematocrit method.

Microhematocrit method

The microhematocrit method is the reference method [107]. Borosilicate or soda-lime glass capillary tubes having a length of 75 mm and an internal diameter of 1.15 mm are recommended. The wall thickness should be 0.20 mm. The requirements for centrifugation are as follows:

- Microhematocrit centrifuge with a rotor radius > 8 cm
- Maximum speed should be reached within 30 sec
- Relative centrifugal force 10,000–15,000 × g at the periphery for 5 min without exceeding a temperature of 45 °C.

The hematocrit is calculated as:

$$\text{Hct} = \frac{\text{Length of red cell column (mm)}}{\text{Length of red cell column plus plasma column (mm)}}$$

Reference Range [67]

Women	35–47%	0.35–0.47
Men	40–52%	0.40–0.52

Red Blood Cell Count

The differentiation of stem cells to erythrocytes begins at the level of the hematopoietic stem cell (CFU-GEMM). From this stage on, all successor cells of erythropoiesis have lost their ability to renew erythropoiesis.

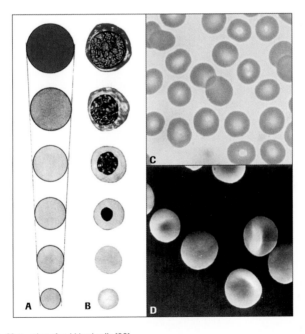

Fig. 55. Maturation of red blood cells [32]

A: cell size and color change depending on degree of maturity
B: loss of chromatin during maturation of red blood cells
C: light microscopic view of erythrocytes
D: electron microscopic view of erythrocytes

Laboratory

As the erythrocytes age, they decrease in volume and deformability and their density increases. Changes in the cell membrane lead to loss of carbohydrates on the cell surface. The normal red cell is removed from the blood stream by the reticuloendothelial system by phagocytosis after 100–120 days.

The hematopoietic stem cell (CFU-GEMM) differentiates into the burst-forming unit erythroid (BFU-E). This stage is followed by the colony-forming unit erythroid (CFU-E). After various divisions, which take several days in vivo, the cells go through a process of typical morphologic and functional differentiation in the process of which they lose their proliferative capacity step by step (Fig. 55).

The red blood cell count (RBC) is a basic examination for the evaluation of disorders of erythropoiesis. Alone it is of little diagnostic value. Only the combination of this parameter with the hematocrit permits differentiation between erythrocytopenia, erythrocytosis or a normal erythrocyte count with reference to the red cell mass of the body.

Reference Range [67]

Women	$4.1–5.1 \times 10^6/\mu L$
Men	$4.5–5.9 \times 10^6/\mu L$

Red Blood Cell Indices

Hematology analyzers calculate the following parameters from the measured red red blood cell count and hemoglobin concentration:
- Mean corpuscular volume (MCV)
- Mean corpuscular hemoglobin (MCH)
- Mean corpuscular hemoglobin concentration (MCHC)

The MCV, MCH, and MCHC are called red cell indices and are used for the description of red cell changes and the differentiation of disturbances of erythropoiesis.

The MCV is expressed in femtoliters (fL, 10^{-15} L or 10^{-9} μL). Hematology analyzers either measure this parameter directly or calculate it according to the following equation:

$$MCV = \frac{\text{Volume of red cells per 1 } \mu\text{L blood}}{\text{Red cells per 1 } \mu\text{L blood}}$$

The mean volume of a single erythrocyte is obtained by the calculation based on the parameters red cell concentration per microliter of blood, and hematocrit:

$$MCV = \frac{\text{Hematocrit (Hct in \%)} \times 10^{-2}}{\text{Red cell count} \times 10^6}[\mu\text{L}] = \frac{\text{Hct in \%} \times 10^{-2} \times 10^9}{\text{Red cell count} \times 10^6}[\text{fL}]$$

e.g.:   Red cells = $5 \times 10^6/\mu\text{L}$
          Hematocrit = 45%

$$MCV = \frac{45 \times 10^{-2} (\times 10^9)}{5 \times 10^6} = \frac{45 \times 10}{5} = 90 \text{ fL}$$

Reference range [67]

Adults	80–96 fL

Note

MCV is reduced in patients with iron deficiency, and it is raised in patients with macrocytic anemias, reticulocytosis, and aplastic anemias.

The MCH is expressed in picograms (pg) and is obtained by calculation from the Hb concentration per microliter and the red cell count per microliter. Hematology analyzers calculate it according to the following equation:

$$MCH = \frac{\mu\text{g Hb in 1 } \mu\text{L blood}}{\text{Red cells per 1 } \mu\text{L blood}}[\text{pg}]$$

$$= \frac{\text{Hb (in g/dL)} \times 10}{\text{Red cells} \times 10^6/\mu\text{L}}[\text{pg}]$$

e.g.:   Red cells = $5 \times 10^6/\mu\text{L}$ blood
          Hemoglobin = 16 g/dL blood = 160 g/L = 160 μg/μL

$$MCH = \frac{160\,\mu g/L}{5 \times 10^6/\mu L} = 32 \times 10^{-6}\,\mu g = 32\,pg$$

Reference Range [67]

Adults	28–33 pg/cell	1.7–2.0 fmol/cell

Note

Hypochromic erythrocytes are present when MCH is less than 28 pg/cell, when Hb is more greatly reduced than red cell count, and in patients with iron deficiency or thalassemia.

Hyperchromic erythrocytes are observed when MCH is over 33 pg, and when the red cell count is more greatly reduced than Hb, or in patients with hyperchromic macrocytosis (e.g., pernicious anemia). The MCHC is expressed in g/dL of red blood cells and is calculated as follows:

$$MCHC = \frac{\text{Hemoglobin concentration (g/dL)}}{\text{Hematocrit (\%)}}$$

e.g.:   Hemoglobin = 15.0 g/dL blood = 150 g/L blood
Hematocrit = 45% = 0.45 L red cells/L blood

$$MCHC = \frac{15 \times 100}{45} = 33\,g\,Hb/dL\ \text{red cells}$$

Reference Range [67]

Adults	33–36 g/dL	20–22 mmol/L

Note

MCV, MCH, and MCHC are important for the classification of anemias and the early detection of processes which can cause anemia.

MCHC is decreased in patients with serious iron deficiency and paramorphias (e.g., thalassemia). MCHC is elevated in patients with spherocytosis and exsiccosis, and in the presence of macro- and microcytic anemias.

Table 45: Classification of the anemias on the basis of MCV, MCH, and MCHC

Red cell indices	Evaluation
MCV reduced MCH reduced MCHC normal, reduced	*Most common form of anemia: microcytic anemia:* Iron deficiency, ACD; disturbance of iron distribution (tumor anemias); deficiency of copper or vitamin B_6; thalassemia.
MCV normal MCH normal MCHC normal	*Normochromic, normocytic anemia:* Non-regenerative anemias, e.g. chronic diseases of the kidneys, endocrine disorders, maldigestion, malabsorption, and malignant tumors.
MCV normal MCH elevated/normal MCHC elevated/normal	*Normocytic, normo/hyperchromic anemia:* Hemolysis, spherocytosis (MCHC elevated).
MCV elevated MCH normal/elevated MCHC normal/decreased	*Macrocytic, hyperchromic anemia:* Folate or vitamin B_{12} deficiency anemia; liver cirrhosis; Alcoholism, MDS (myelodisplastic syndrome).

Determination of the MCV is used for the diagnostically important distinction between normocytic, microcytic, and macrocytic anemias. The MCV is dependent on the hydration of the red cells and on the red cell distribution width in the plasma. In the majority of the anemias the MCH correlates with the MCV. Microcytic anemias correspond to hypochromic anemias, normocytic to normochromic anemias.

Reticulocyte Count

Reticulocytes are a transitional form between the nucleated erythroblast and the anucleate mature erythrocyte. The reticulocyte is a very young erythrocyte which contains precipitated nucleic acids after supravital staining. For identification as a reticulocyte the cell must contain two or more clumps or blue-stained granules which must be visible microscopically without fine-focusing of the cell.

Reticulocytes are purged from the bone marrow into the peripheral blood approximately 18–36 hours before their final maturation. As such, they represent a system for the detection of the real-time status of erythropoiesis. Changes in the reticulocyte concentration in the blood correlate with the release of immature precursor stages, but not with the

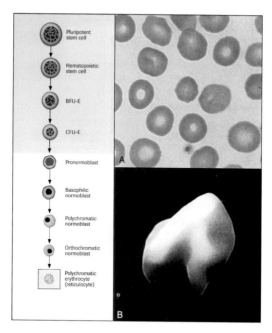

Fig. 56: Degrees of maturation of reticulocytes [32]
      A: polychromatic erythrocytes (reticulocytes)
      B: electron-microscopic image of a reticulocyte

actual formation of blood cells in the bone marrow [32]. The determination of the reticulocyte count is used for:

- Determination of the bone marrow activity needed for the renewal of RBCs consumed in the peripheral blood (e.g., suspicious of intravascular hemolysis and blood loss).
- Detection of disturbances in RBC formation as a result of deficiencies of certain substances and monitoring the response to therapy in deficiency anemias, e.g. iron, copper, vitamin B_6, vitamin B_{12}, and folate deficiency.
- Evaluation of erythropoiesis after erythropoietin administration. It has been proposed that response to treatment with erythropoietin can be detected by measuring hemoglobin and reticulocyte count 4 weeks after starting therapy. An increase in Hb concentration by 1 g/dL or

reticulocyte concentration by $>40 \times 10^9/L$ is reportedly indicative of patient response.
- Assessment of the marrow's ability to regenerate after cytotoxic or myeloablative therapy and bone marrow transplantation.

The reticulocyte count is expressed either as a percentage (number of reticulocytes/100 mature red blood cells) or as an absolute cell count (reticulocytes/µL).

Reference Range [67]

Adults	5–15‰	50,000–100,000/µL

The reticulocyte count expressed as percentage can be falsely elevated if the number of mature red blood cells is low, e.g., in patients with anemia. A number of correction formulas have been recommended in order to make the clinical interpretation of reticulocyte counts easier to understand.

The reticulocyte count expressed as per cent can be elevated either due to true replication of reticulocytes in the circulating blood or by a

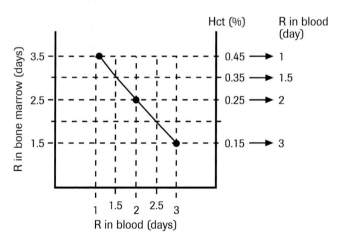

Fig. 57: Maturation (bone marrow) and residence time (blood) of reticulocytes (R) and relation to hematocrit (Hct)

lower percentage of mature erythrocytes. In the case of anemia, the reticulocyte count requires a hematocrit-dependent correction expressed as the reticulocyte index.

Reticulocyte index

The percentage of reticulocytes can increase due to higher reticulocyte counts or falling RBC counts. The correction can be performed based on the patient's hematocrit (Hct) with reference to an ideal Hct of 0.45. This correction is recommended in patients with anemias:

$$\text{Reticulocyte index (RI): RI} = \text{reticulocytes (\%)} \times \frac{\text{Hct (patient)}}{0.45}$$

Reticulocyte production index (RPI)

For purposes of clinical assessment, the reticulocyte production index (RPI) should be determined as well.

Under normal conditions, reticulocytes become mature in the bone marrow in 3.5 days, and in 1 day while circulating in the blood.

In states of intensive erythropoietic stress, e.g., if hematocrit (Hct) drops, the maturation time of these "stress" reticulocytes in the bone marrow can be reduced to 1.5 days and, on balance, it increases in the blood. Since reticulocytes are excreted in immature stages, the number of circulating reticulocytes can increase markedly as a result without the erythropoietic activity being elevated.

The maturation time of reticulocytes in the bone marrow behaves in proportion to the Hct, i.e., it drops with Hct and, correspondingly, the maturation time in blood increases (Table 46, Fig. 57). The reticulocyte count corrected for the respective maturation time and normal Hct of 0.45 is called the Reticulocyte Production Index (RPI).

Table 46: Hematocrit-dependent dwell time of reticulocytes in blood. According to [71]

Hematocrit	Residence time of reticulocytes in blood (shift)
45%	1 Day
35%	1.5 Days
25%	2 Days
15%	2.5 Days

Reticulocyte Production Index (RPI)
$RPI = \dfrac{\text{Reticulocyte count in \%}}{\text{Maturation time in blood in days}} \times \dfrac{\text{Hct (patient)}}{0.45 \text{ (ideal Hct)}}$

Example: Hct = 25%, R = 20%, maturation time in blood: 2 days

$$RPI = \frac{20 \times 0.25}{2 \times 0.45} = 5.5$$

In this case, erythrocyte production is increased 5.5-fold.

The reticulocyte production index is normally 1 when erythrocyte formation and degradation are in balance. In the presence of anemia, an index value of > 2 indicates adequate renewal. Depending on the severity of the anemia, an RPI value of < 2 indicates hypoplasia or ineffective erythropoiesis. A bone marrow swab must also be obtained in order to perform a quantitative and qualitative assessment of erythropoiesis for a clinical assessment of the RPI.

In the case of normal, i.e., effective erythropoiesis, the number of reticulocytes correlates directly with the renewal of red cell formation. Under an intensified effect of erythropoietin, reticulocyte maturation is shifted. The physiologic maturation time of reticulocytes is four days, three of which are spent in the bone marrow and one in the peripheral blood. The assessment of reticulocyte counts in clinical practice is based on this behavior. In the presence of anemia and depending on the hematocrit, maturation of the reticulocytes is moved to the peripheral blood with a correspondingly longer presence in the circulating blood. The changed residence time of the reticulocytes in the peripheral blood is called the "shift". The number of reticulocytes determined in the blood must be reduced by this number for making a clinical statement about the actual renewal ability of erythropoiesis. Without this shift correction, the reticulocyte values determined would be too high. The real numbers are calculated independence on the hematocrit with the aid of the reticulocyte production index.

The RPI can be useful in clarifying the causes of anemia. An RPI > 2.0 is associated with chronic hemolysis, bleeding or an effective therapy of existing anemia. Indices < 2.0 are associated with marrow insufficiency or ineffective erythropoiesis such as vitamin B_{12} or folic acid deficiency anemias.

The automated reticulocyte count ensures high counting precision. In addition, the maturation index (RNA content) and the cell indices (volume and Hb content) of the reticulocytes are determined. As a result, their counting and analytical testing are gaining in clinical significance and acceptance for various diagnostic issues, especially in terms of the count results in the low range.

Hemoglobin Content of Reticulocytes

Many studies in the differentiation of anemias and for monitoring erythropoietin therapy demonstrated that the hemoglobin content of the reticulocytes (Ret-Hb) is an early indicator of iron-deficient erythropoiesis even when serum ferritin or transferrin saturation is still normal [28]. The Ret-Hb increases markedly in dialysis patients who receive i.v. iron simultaneously with EPO during therapy. In the field of pediatrics as well, Ret-Hb has proven to be a good indicator for iron deficiency in children [28]. Ret-Hb can be provided using modern hematology systems. The normal range for Ret-Hb is 28–35 pg per reticulocyte.

Erythrocyte Ferritin

In a few studies, erythrocyte ferritin is proposed in place of serum ferritin as a parameter for anemia patients with chronic disease. The determination is not as easy to perform as for serum ferritin, and erythrocyte ferritin responds very late to dynamic changes. If, in the case of iron deficiency, practically the entire population of red blood cells has been replaced with erythrocytes having a low Hb content, erythrocyte ferritin first drops to pathologically low values. The determination of erythrocyte ferritin has not become part of daily routine testing.

Zinc Protoporphyrin

The measurement of zinc protoporphyrin (ZPP) is a rapid method, but it requires a special hematofluorimeter. An elevated ZPP value in untreated blood is non-specific.

False positive values are observed primarily in patients with liver disease, infectious disease, and malignomas. Hastka found greatly elevated ZPP values caused by drug interferences [63]. Elevated values of bilirubin cause interference as well, as in the presence of cholestase, hepatitis or hemolytic anemias. ZPP contents that were apparently elevated were also found in patients with chronic kidney disease.

An apparently elevated ZPP concentration in the blood is caused by fluorescence interference of drugs, bilirubin or – as in the case of kidney disease – in non-dialyzable, high molecular-weight plasma components. The yellow, red or brown intrinsic colors are described as particularly disturbing [63]. On the other hand, ZPP values that are too low are measured when blood is stored. This is due to the shift in the absorbance spectrum of deoxygenated hemoglobin.

Before measuring ZPP in hematofluorimeters, it is therefore recommended that the red cells be washed. This reduces ZPP normal values from 50 to 32 µmol/mol heme. Although the ZPP determination increases in specificity as a result, the washing procedure must be performed manually. This cancels out the advantage of the rapid automated ZPP determination.

Tests for the Diagnosis of Chronic Inflammation

Inflammation can be detected using the following tests:
- Erythrocyte sedimentation rate (ESR)
- Quantitative determination of C-reactive protein (CRP) and/or serum amyloid A protein (SAA)
- Interleukin-6 (IL-6), Interleukin-8 (IL-8), and Tumor Necrosis factor-α (TNF-α) determination
- Differential blood count and leukocyte count.

Laboratory

Erythrocyte Sedimentation Rate

Method

A citrated blood sample is aspirated into a glass or plastic pipette with millimeter graduation up to the 200 mm mark. The pipette remains in an upright position and the sedimentation of red cells is read off in mm after one hour. The performance of the method follows an approved guideline.

Reference Range [67]

Age	<50 years	>50 years
Women	<25 mm/h	<30 mm/h
Men	<15 mm/h	<20 mm/h

In comparison to the quantitative determination of an acute phase protein, e.g. CRP, the Erythrocyte Sedimentation Rate (ESR) is also raised by an increase in the concentration of immunoglobulins, immune complexes, and other proteins. It therefore covers a broader spectrum of diseases than CRP. In the case of chronic inflammatory disease, e.g. in SLE (systemic lupus erythrematodes), in which CRP is often normal or only slightly elevated, and for monitoring in patients with these diseases, the ESR is therefore a better indicator of the inflammatory process.

C-Reactive Protein

C-reactive protein (CRP) is the classic acute phase protein that is released in response to an inflammatory reaction. It is synthesized in the liver.

CRP is composed of five identical, non-glycosylated subunits each comprising a single polypeptide chain of 206 amino acid residues with a molecular mass of 23,000 daltons. The characteristic structure places CRP in the family of pentraxins (calcium-binding proteins with immune defense properties).

CRP synthesis increases rapidly following induction by the inflammatory cytokines like IL-6. At the peak of an acute phase response, as much as 20% of the protein synthesizing capacity of the liver may be engaged in its synthesis. Increased serum CRP levels are always an indicator of inflammation. However, in Hodgkin's disease, the kidney carcinoma cells can also secrete inflammatory cytokines and which prompt an acute phase response that induces fever and raised serum concentrations of CRP.

CRP determination is used
- for confirmation of the presence of acute organic disease such as cardiac infarction, deep vein thrombosis and infections; chronic conditions such as malignant tumors, rheumatic diseases, and inflammatory bowel disease. For diagnosis and monitoring of infections when microbiologic testing is too slow or impossible.
- as an aid in the management of rheumatic diseases.
- for rapid establishment of the optimum anti-inflammatory therapy and the determination of the minimal effective dose [112].

CRP is the most sensitive of the acute phase proteins which can be readily measured in the routine laboratory. At present there are no clear indications for the determination of other acute phase proteins.

Methods
Various automated nephelometric and turbidimetric assays for CRP determination are available. The least measurable dose should be at least 5 mg/L and it should be lower for the diagnosis of newborns.

Reference range [67]

Adults	< 0.5 mg/dL	< 5 mg/L

Interleukin-6

The determination of Interleukin-6 (IL-6) in plasma – which is the preferred specimen – is well suited as prognostic parameter in sepsis, trauma, and heart failure, and for early diagnosis of neonatal sepsis. Its use is less well established for determining the disease activity in patients with chronic inflammatory processes, e.g. rheumathoid arthritis.

An elevated IL-6 concentration does not allow to reach any differential diagnostic conclusion. Instead, it is just an indicator of an ongoing inflammatory response from various causes [146].

Laboratory

Important considerations for accurate results are an appropriate preanalysis (separation of plasma and cells within 2 h; storage for >1 d at −20 °C; prolonged storage at −70°C) and the use of tests that are standardized against WHO standards. Different immunoassay kits are available. The results, however, are only of limited comparability.

Reference Range [67]

Serum or plasma	<10 ng/L

Adequately evaluated reference intervals for urine and other body fluids do not exist. IL-6 concentrations >1000 ng/L are in general associated with a high mortality.

Interleukin-8

The determination of Interleukin-8 (IL-8) in plasma – which is the preferred specimen – is suitable not only as a prognostic parameter in sepsis, trauma, and heart failure but also in the early diagnosis of neonatal sepsis.

An elevated IL-8 concentration does not allow any differential diagnostic conclusions to be reached. Instead, it is just an indicator of an ongoing inflammatory response of various causes [146]. During the assessment, it must be taken into account that IL-8 can be produced by immune cells, i.e. mainly monocytes, macrophages, as well as by nonimmune cells, e.g. endothelial or epithelial cells.

Important considerations for accurate results are an appropriate preanalysis (separation of plasma and cells within 2 h; storage for >1 d at − 20°C; prolonged storage at −70°C) and the use of tests that are standardized against WHO standards. Different enzyme immunoassay kits are available. The results, however, are only of limited comparability.

Reference Range [13]

Females, 4–12 yr	0.56–5.33 ng/L
Males, 4–12 yr	0.57–4.58 ng/L
Females/Males, 13–17 yr	0.56–5.54 ng/L
Females/Males, 18–39 yr	0.56–3.80 ng/L
Females/Males, 44–55 yr	0.56–7.52 ng/L

Laboratory

IL-8 concentrations of > 500 ng/L are generally associated with high mortality.

Tumor Necrosis Factor-α

Tumor Necrosis Factor-α (TNF-α) in plasma is a marker for an ongoing inflammatory response of various causes [146]. Elevated TNF- α levels indicate an excessive and/or prolonged inflammatory reaction with systemic manifestation.

Important considerations for accurate results are an appropriate pre-analysis (separation of plasma and cells within 2 h; storage for > 1 d at –20 °C; prolonged storage at –70°C) and the use of tests that are standardized against WHO standards. Different enzyme immunoassay kits and bioassays are available. Some assays detect the biologically active trimer of TNF-α, while other tests also detect biologically inactive monomers and other degradation products in addition to the trimer i.e., they detect total TNF-α. Therefore, the results obtained with the different tests are hardly comparable.

Reference Range [146]

Total TNF-α	< 20 ng/L
Bioactive TNF-α	< 5 ng/L

Adequately evaluated reference ranges in other body fluids are not available.

References

[1] Aapro MS and Link H (2009) September 2007 update on EORT guidelines and anemia managent with erythropoiesis-stimulating agents. Oncologist 13 (suppl): 33–36

[2] Aisen P (1998) Transferrin, the transferrin receptor, and the uptake of iron by cells. In: Siegel S and Siegel H (eds) Metal ions in biological systems, Vol. 35. Marcel Dekker, New York, pp 585–631

[3] Albertini A, Arosio P, Chiancone E and Drysdale J (eds) (1984) Ferritins and isoferritins as biochemical markers. Elsevier, Amsterdam NewYork Oxford

[4] Alford CE, King TTE and Campell PA (1991) Role of transferrin, transferrin receptors and iron in macrophage listericidal activity. J Med 174: 459–466

[5] Andrews NC (1999) Disorders of iron metabolism. N Engl J Med 341: 1986–1995

[6] Arnett FC, Edworthy SM, Bloch DA, McShane DJ, Fries JF, Cooper NS, et al. (1988) The American Rheumatism Association 1987 revised criteria for the classification of rheumatoid arthritis. Arthritis Rheum 31: 315–324

[7] Arosio P, Levi S, Gabri E, et al. (1984) Heterogeneity of ferritin II: immunological aspects. In: Albertini A, Arosio P, Chiancone E and Drysdale J (eds) Ferritins and isoferritins as biochemical markers. Elsevier, Amsterdam New York Oxford, pp 33–47

[8] Ascherio A, Rimm EB, Giovanucci E, Willet WC and Stampfer MJ (2001) Blood donation and risk of coronary heart disease. Circulation 103: 52–57

[9] Ascherio A, Rimm EB, Giovanucci E and Stampfer MJ (1994) Dietary iron intake and risk of coronary disease among men. Circulation 89: 969–974

[10] Ashrafian H (2003) Hepcidin: the missing link between hemochromatosis and infections. Infect Immun 71: 6693–6700

[11] Baker EN and Lindley PF (1992) New perspectives on the structure and function of transferrin. J Inorg Biochem 47: 147–160

[12] Barakat RM and Ekins RP (1961) Assay of vitamin B12 in blood. A simple method. Lancet 2: 25–26

[13] Barrahmoune H, Lamont JU, Herbeth B, FitzGerald PS and Visvikis-Siest S (2006) Biological determinants of and reference

values for plasma interleukin-8, monocyte chemoattractant protein-I, epidermal growth factor, and vascular endothelial growth factor: results from the STANISLAS cohort. Clin Chem 52: 504–510

[14] Baynes RD (1994) Iron deficiency. In: Brock JH, Halliday JW, Pippard MJ and Powell LW (eds) Iron metabolism in health and disease. WB Saunders Co, London, pp 189–198

[15] Baynes RD (1996) Assessment of iron status. Clin Biochem 29: 209–215

[16] Begemann H and Rastetter J (1993) Klinische Haematologie, [4] Aufl. Thieme, Stuttgart-New York

[17] Beguin Y (1998) Prediction of response to treatment with recombinant human erythropoietin in anemia associated with cancer. Med Oncol 15 (Suppl 1): 38–46

[18] Beguin Y (1992) The soluble transferrin receptor: biological aspects and clinical usefulness as quantitative measure of erythropoiesis. Haematologica 77: 1–10

[19] Beguin Y, Clemons GK, Pootrakul P and Fillet G (1993) Quantitative asessment of erythropoiesis and functional classification of anemia based on measurement of serum transferrin receptor and erythropoietin. Blood 81: 1067–1076

[20] Beguin Y (2003) Soluble transferrin receptor for the evaluation of erythropoisis and iron status. Clin Chim Acta 329: 9–22

[21] Besarab A, Bolton WK, Browne JK, Egrie JC, Nissenson AR, Okamato DM et al. (1998) The effect of normal as compared with low hematocrit values in patients with cardiac disease who are receiving hemodialysis and Erythropoietin. N Engl J Med 339: 584–590

[22] Beutler E (1997) Genetic irony beyond haemochromatosis: clinical effects of HLA-H mutations. Lancet 349: 296–297

[23] Bobbio-Pallavicini F, Verde G, Spriano B, Losi R, Bosatra MG and Brasch A (1989) Body iron status in critically ill patients: significance of serum ferritin. Int Care Med 15: 171–178

[24] Boelaert JR, Weinberg GA and Weinberg ED (1996) Altered iron metabolism in HIV infection: Mechanisms, possible consequences and proposals for management. Inf Dis Agents 5: 36–46

[25] Bothwell TH, Baynes RD, MacFarlane BJ and MacPhail AP (1989) Nutritional iron requirements and food iron absorption. J Intern Med 226: 357–365

[26] Brock JH (1994) Iron in infection, immunity, inflammation and neoplasia. In: Brock JH, Halliday JW, Pippard MJ, Powell LW and London WB (eds) Iron metabolism in health and disease. Saunders, London, pp 353–389

[27] Brouwer DAJ, Welten HTME, Reijngoud DJ, van Doormaal JJ and Muskiet FAJ (1998) Plasma folic acid cutoff value, derived from its relationship with homocyst(e)ine. Clin Chem 44: 1545–1550

[28] Brugnara C (2000) Reticulocyte cellular indices: a new approach in the diagnosis of anemias and monitoring of erythropoietic function. Critical Rev in Clin Lab Sci 37: 93–130

[29] Bunn HF (1991) Anemia associated with chronic disorders. In: Harrison's principles of internal medicine, 12th ed. McGraw-Hill, New York, pp 1529–1531

[30] Burmester G (1998) Taschenatlas der Immunologie: Grundlagen, Labor; Klinik. Thieme, Stuttgart, New York

[31] Burns DL and Pomposelli JJ (1999) Toxicity of parenteral iron dextran therapy. Kid Int 55 (Suppl 69): 119–124

[32] Carr H and Rodak BF (1999) Clinical hematology atlas. WB Saunders, Philadelphia

[33] Carmel R (1997) Cobalamin, the stomach and aging. Am J Clin Nutr 66: 750–759

[34] Cazzola M, Mercuriali F and Brugnara C (1997) Use of recombinant human erythropoietin outside the setting of uraemia. Blood 89: 4248–4267

[35] Cazzola M, Ponchio L, de Benedetti F, Ravelli A, Rosti V, Beguin Y, et al. (1996) Defective iron supply for erythropoiesis and adequate endogenous erythropoietin production in anemia associated with systemic onset invenile chronic arthritis. Blood 87: 4824–4830

[36] Cazzola M, Ponchio L, Pedrotti C, Farina G, Cerani P, Lucotti C, et al. (1996) Prediction to response of recombinant human erythropoietin (rh-EPO) in anaemia of malignancy. Haematologica 81: 434–441

[37] Cheung W, Minton N, Gunawardena K and Frey K (2001) The pharmacokinetics and pharmacodynamics of epoietin alfa once weekly versus 3 times weekly. Eur J Clin Pharmacol 57: 411–418

[38] Cook JD, Skikne BS and Baynes RD (1993) Serum transferrin receptor. Ann Rev Med 44: 63–74

[39] Cook JD, Skikne BS and Baynes RD (1986) Estimates of iron sufficiency in the US population. Blood 68: 726–731

[40] Corti MC, Gaziano M and Hennekeus CH (1997) Iron status and risk of cardiovascular disease. Ann Epidemiol 7: 62–68

[41] Dallalio G, Fleury T and Means RT (2003) Serum hepcidin in clinical specimens. Brit J Haematol 122: 996–1000

[42] De Jong G, von Dijk IP and van Eijk HG (1990) The biology of transferrin. Clin Chim Acta 190: 1–46

[43] De Sousa M, Reimao R, Porto G, Grady RW, Hilgartner MW and Giardina P (1992) Iron and lymphocytes: reciprocal regulatory interactions. Curr Stud Hematol Blood Transf 58: 171–177

[44] Pointner H (1992) Folsäure-Resorptionstest. In: Deutsch E, Geyer G and Wenger R (eds) Laboratoriumsdiagnostik. Karger, Basel, pp 91–93

[45] Dietzfelbinger H (1993) Korpuskuläre hamolytische Anämien. In: Begemann H und Rastetter J (Hrsg) Klinische Haematologie, 4. Aufl. Thieme, Stuttgart-New York, S 248–252

[46] Dinant JC, de Kock CA and van Wersch JWJ (1995) Diagnostic value of C-reactive protein measurement does not justify replacement of the erythrocyte sedimentation rate in daily general practice. Eur J Clin Invest 25: 353–359

[47] Egrie JC, Dwyer E, Lykos M, Hitz A and Browne JK (1997) Novel erythropoiesis stimulating protein (NESP) has a longer serum half-life and greater in vitro biological activity compared to recombinant human erythropoietin (rHU EPO). Blood 90: 56 A (abstract)

[48] Erslev AJ (1991) Erythropoietin. New Engl J Med 324: 1339–1344

[49] Eschbach JW, Haley NR and Adamson JW (1990) The anemia of chronic renal failure: pathophysiology and effects of recombinant erythropoietin. Contrib Nephrol 78: 24–37

[50] Feelders RA, Kuiper-Kramer EPA and van Eijk HG (1999) Structure, function and clinical significance of transferrin receptors. Clin Chem Lab Med 37: 1–10

[51] Ferguson BJ, Skikne BS, Simpson KM, Baynes RD and Cook JD (1992) Serum transferrin receptor distinguishes the anemia of chronic disease from iron deficiency anemia. J Lab Clin Med 19: 385–390

[52] Fisher JW (2003) Erythropoietin. Erythropoietin: physiology and pharmacology update. Exp Biol Med 228: 1–14

[53] Folkman J (1997) Addressing tumor blood vessels. Nat Biotechnol 15: 110–115

[54] Frishman WH (1998) Biologic markers as predictors of cardiovascular disease. Am J Med 104: 18s–27s

[55] Gabrilove JL, Cleeland CS, Livingston RB, et al. (2001) Clinical evaluation of once-weekly dosing of epoietin Alfa in chemotherapy patients: improvements in hemoglobin and quality of life are similar to three-times-weekly dosing. J Clin Oncol 19: 2875–2882

[56] Gargano G, Polignano G, De Lena M, Brandi M, Lorusso V and Fanizza G (1999) The utility of a growth factor: rHU-EPO as a treatment for pre-operative autologous blood donation in gynaecological tumor surgery. Int J Oncol 4 (1): 157–160

[57] Goldberg MA, Dunning SP and Bunn HF (1988) Regulation of the erythropoietin gene: evidence, that the oxygen sensor is a hemo protein. Science 24w: 1412–1415

[58] Graf H, Lacombe JL, Braun J, Gomes da Costa AA and on behalf of the European/Australian NESP 970 290 study group (2000) Novel erythropoiesis stimulating protein (NESP) effectively maintains hemoglobin (Hgb) when administered at a reduced dose frequency compared with recombinant human erythropoietin (r-HuEPO) in dialysis patients. J Am Soc Nephrol 11: A1317

[59] Graziadei I, Gaggl S, Kaserbacher R, Braunsteiner H and Vogl W (1994) The acute phase protein alpha-1 antitrypsin inhibits growth and proliferation on human early erythroid progenitor cells and of human erythroleucemic cells by interfering with transferrin iron uptake. Blood 83: 260–268

[60] Greendyke RM, Sharma K and Gifford FR (1994) Serum levels of erythropoietin and selected cytokines in patients with anemia of chronic disease. Am Clin Path 101: 338–341

[61] Grützmacher P, Ehmer B, Messinger D, et al. (1991) Therapy with recombinant human Erythropoietin (rEPO) in hemodialysis patients with transfusion dependent anemia. Report of a European multicenter trial. Nephrologia 11: 58–65

[62] Gunshin H, Mackenzie B, Berger UV, et al. (1997) Cloning and characterization of a mammalian proton-coupled metal-ion transporter. Nature 388: 482–488

[63] Hastka J, Lasserre JJ, Schwarzbeck A, Strauch M and Hehlmann R (1992) Washing erythrocyte to remove interferents in measurements of zinc protoporphyrin by front-face hematofluorometry. Clin Chem 11: 2184–2189

[64] Haupt H and Baudner S (1990) Chemie und klinische Bedeutung der Human Plasma Proteine. Behring Institut Mitteilungen 86: 1–66

[65] Haverkate F, Thompson SG, Pyke SD, Gallimore JR and Pepys MB (1997) Production of C-reactive protein and risk of coronary events in stable and unstable angina. European Concerted Action on Thrombosis and Disabilities Angina Pectoris Study Group. Lancet 349: 462–466

[66] Heidelberger M and Kendall FE (1935) The precipitin reaction between type III pneumococcus polysaccharide and homologous antibody III. A quantitative study and theory of the reaction mechanism. J Exp Med 61: 563–591

[67] Heil W and Ehrhardt V (2008) Reference ranges for adults and children, 9th edn. Roche Diagnostics Ltd., Rotkreuz, Switzerland

[68] Heinrich HC (1986) Bioverfügbarkeit und therapeutische Wirksamkeit oraler Eisen (2)- und (3) Praparate. Schweiz. Apotheker-Zeitung 22: 1231–1256

[69] Henke M, Guttenberger R, Barke A, Pajonk F, Potter R and Frommhold H (1999) Erythropoietin for patients undergoing radiotherapy: a pilot study. Radiother Oncol 502: 185–190

[70] Herrmann W, Schorr H, Purschwitz K, Rassoul F and Richter V (2001) Total homocysteine, vitamin B12, and total antioxidant status in vegetarians. Clin Chem 47: 1094–1101

[71] Hillman RS and Finch CA (1985) Red cell manual, 5th edn. Davis, Philadelphia

[72] Hörl WH, Cavill I, Macdougall IC, Schaefer RM and Sunder-Plassmann G (1996) How to diagnose and correct iron deficiency during rhEPO therapy, a consensus report. Nephrol Dial Transplant 11: 246–250

[73] Huebers HA, Beguin Y, Pootrakne P, Einspahr D and Finch CA (1990) Intact transferrin receptors in human plasma and their relation to erythropoiesis. Blood 75: 102–107

[74] http://www.biocarta.com/pathfiles/h_TH1TH2Pathway.asp

[75] International Committee for Standardisation in Haematology (1988) Recommendations for measurement of serum iron in blood. Int J Hematol 6: 107–111

[76] Jacobs A, Hodgetts J and Hoy TG (1984) Functional aspects of isoferritins. In: Albertini A, Arosio P, Chiancone E and Drysdale J (eds) Ferritins and isoferritins as biochemical markers. Elsevier, Amsterdam New York Oxford, pp 113–127

[77] Jiang R, Manson JE, Meigs JB, Ma J, Rifai N and Hu FB (2004) Body iron stores in relation to risk of type 2 diabetes in apparently healthy women. JAMA 291: 711–717

[78] Johnson AM (1996) Other proteins: ceruloplasmin. In: Ritchie RF and Navolotskaia O (eds) Serum proteins in clinical medicine. Foundation for Blood Research, Scarborough, MA

[79] Jouanolle AM, Gandon G, Jézéquel P, Blayau M, et al. (1996) Haemochromatosis and HLA-H. Nature Genet 14: 251–252

[80] Kaltwasser JP, Kessler U, Gottschalk R, Stucki G and Moller B (2001) Effect of rHU-erythropoietin and i.v. iron on anaemia and disease activity in rheumatoid arthritis. J Rheumatol 28: 2430–2437

[81] Kiechl S, Willeit J, Egger G, et al. (1997) Body iron stores and the risk of carotid atherosclerosis: prospective results from the Bruneck Study. Circulation 96: 3300–3307

[82] Knekt P, Reunanen A, Takkunen H, Aromaa A, Heliövaara M and Hakuunen T (1994) Body iron stores and the risk of cancer. Int J Cancer 56: 379–382

[83] Kolbe-Busch S, Lotz J, Hafner G, Blanckaert J, Claeys G, Togni G, Carlsen J, Röddiger R and Thomas L (2002) Multicenter evaluation of a fully mechanized soluble transferrin receptor assay on the Hitachi and COBAS INTEGRA analyzers and determination of reference ranges. Clin Chem Lab Med 40: 529–536

[84] Kubasik NP, Ricotta M and Sine HE (1980) Comercially supplied binders for plasmacobalamin (vitamin B_{12}) analysis – "purified" intrinsic factor, "cobinamide"-blocked R-protein binder, and non-purified intrinsic factor-R-protein binder – compared to microbiological assay. Clin Chem 26: 598–600

[85] Leedman PJ, Stein AR, Chin WW and Rogers JT (1996) Thyroid hormone modulates the interaction between iron regulatory proteins and the ferritin mRNA iron responsive element. J Biol Chem 271: 12017–12023

[86] Lejeune FJ, Rüegg C and Liénard D (1998) Clinical applications on TNF-alpha in cancer. Curr Opin Immunol 10: 573–580

[87] Leon P, Jimence M, Barona P and Sierrasesumaga L (1998) Recombinant human erythropoietin for the treatment of anemia in children with solid malignant tumors. Med Pediatr Oncol 30 (2): 110–116

[88] Lichtman MA (2001) William's hematology, 6th edn. McGraw-Hill, New York

[89] Linkesch W (1986) Ferritin bei malignen Erkrankungen. Springer, Wien-NewYork

[90] Linker CA (2009) Blood disorders. In: McPhee SJ and Papadakis MA (eds) Current medical diagnosis and treatment, 48th edn. McGraw-Hill, New York, pp 427–464

[91] Littlewood TJ, Bajetta E, Nortier JW, Vercammen E and Rapoport B (2001) Epoetin Alfa Study Group: effects of epoetin alfa on hematologic parameters and quality of life in cancer patients receiving nonplatinum chemotherapy: results of a randomized, doubleblind, placebo-controlled trial. J Clin Oncol 19: 2865–2874

[92] Loher F and Endress S (2001) Suppression of synthesis of tumor necrosis factor. Internist 42: 28–34

[93] Ludwig H, Fritz E, Leitgeb C, Pecherstorfer M, Samonigg H and Schuster J (1994) Prediction of response to erythropoietin treatment in chronic anemia of cancer. Blood 84: 1056–1063

[94] MacDougall IC, Gray SJ, Elston O, Breen C, Jenkins B, Browne J and Egrie J (1999) Pharmaco-kinetics of novel erythropoiesis stimulating protein compared with erythropoietin alfa in dialysis patients. J Am Soc Nephrol 10: 2392–2395

[95] Macdougall IC and Eckart K (2006) Novel strategies for stimulating erythropoiesis and potential new treatments for anemia. Lancet 368: 947–953

[96] Macdougall IC, Robson R, Oparna S, et al. (2006) Pharmacokinetics and pharmacodynamics of intravenous and subccoutaneous erythropoietin receptor activator (C.E.R.A.) in patients with chronic kidney disease. Clin J Am Soc Nephrol 1: 1211–1215

[97] Maini RN, Breedveld FC, Kalden JR, Smolen JS, Davis D, Macfarlane JD, et al. (1998) Therapeutic efficacy of multiple intravenous infusions of anti-tumor necrosis factor monoclonal antibody combined with low-dose weekly methotrexate in rheumatoid arthritis. Arthritis Rheum 41: 1552–1563

[98] Mangold C (1998) The causes and prognostic significance of low hemoglobin levels in tumor patients. Strahlenther Onkol 174 (suppl 4): 17–19

[99] Mantovani G, Ghiani M, Curreli L, Maccio A, Massa D, Succu G, et al. (1999) Assessment of the efficacy of two dosages and schedules of human recombinant erythropoietin in prevention and correction of cisplatin induced anemia in cancer patients. Oncol Rep 6: 421–426

[100] Massey AC (1992) Microcytic anemia. Differential diagnosis and management of iron deficient anemia. Med Clin North Am 76: 549–566

[101] Mast AE, Blinder MA, Gronowski AM, Chumley C, Scott MG, et al. (1998) Clinical utility of the soluble transferrin receptor and comparison with serum ferritin in several populations. Clin Chem 44: 45–51

[102] Means RT (1995) Pathogenesis of the anemia of chronic disease: A cytokine mediated anemia. Stem Cells (Dayt) 13: 32–37

[103] Menacci A, Cenci E, Boelaert JR, et al. (1997) Iron overload alters T helper cell responses to Candida albicans in mice. J Infect Dis 175: 1467–1476

[104] Mercuriali F, Gualtieri G, Sinigaglia L, et al. (1994) Use of recombinant human erythropoietin to assist autologous blood donation by anemic rheumatiod arthritis patients undergoing major orthopedic surgery. Transfusion 34: 501–506

[105] Moldawer LL and Copeland EM (1997) Proinflammatory cytokines, nutritional support, and the cachexia syndrome: interactions and therapeutic options. Cancer 79: 1828–1839

[106] Mutane J, Piug-Parellada P and Mitjavila MT (1995) Iron metabolism and oxidative stress during acute and chronic phases of experimental inflammation. Effect of iron dextran and desferoxamine. J Lab Clin Med 126: 435–443

[107] NCCLS (1993) Procedure for determining packed cell volume by the microhematocrit method, 2nd edn.; approved standard. NCCLS Document H7 – A2, Vol. 13, no. 9. Villanova: NCCLS

[108] Nowrousian MR (2002) Pathophysiology of cancer-related anemia. In: Nowrousian MR (ed) Recombinant human erythropoietin in clinical oncology: scientific and clinical aspects of anemia in cancer. Springer Medicine, New York, pp 13–34

[109] Park JE, Lentner MC, Zimmermann RN, et al. (1999) Fibroblast activation protein, a dual specificity serine protease expressed in reactive human tumor stromal fibroblasts. J Biol Chem 274: 36505–36512

[110] Paruta S and Hörl WH (1999) Iron and infection. Kidney Int 55: 125–130

[111] Peeters HRM, Jongen-Lavrencic M and Bakker CH (1999) Recombinant human Erythropoetin improves health-related quality of life in patients with rheumatoid arthritis and anaemia of chronic disease; utility measures correlate strongly with disease activity measures. Rheumatol Int 18: 201–206

[112] Pepys MB (1995) The acute phase response and C-reactive protein. In: Weatherall DJ, Kuller LH, Tracy RP, Shaten J and Meilahn EN (eds) Oxford textbook of medicine, 3rd edn. Oxford University Press, Oxford, England, pp 1527–1533

[113] Pietranglo A (2004) Hereditary hemochromatosis – a new look at an old disease. N Engl J Med 350: 2383–2397

[114] Pincus T, Olsen NJ, Russell IJ, et al. (1990) Multicenter study of recombinant human Erythropoietin in correction of anemia in rheumatoid arthritis. Am J Med 89: 161–168

[115] Ponka P (1999) Cellular iron metabolism. Kidney Int 55 (Suppl 69): S2–S11

[116] Ponka P, Beaumont C and Richardson R (1998) Function and regulation of transferrin and ferritin. Semin Hematol 35: 35–54

[117] Punnonen K, Irjala K and Rajamaki A (1994) Iron deficiency anemia is associated with high concentrations of transferrin receptor in serum. Clin Chem 40: 774–776

[118] Qvist N, Boesby S, Wolff B and Hansen CP (1999) Recombinant human erythropoietin and hemoglobin concentrations at operation and during the postoperative period. World J Surg 23: 30–35

[119] Rauramaa R, Väisänen S, Mercuri M, Rankinen T, Penttilä I and Bond MG (1994) Association of risk factors and body iron status to carotid atherosclerosis in middle aged eastern Finnish men. Eur Heart J 15: 1020–1027

[120] Refsum H, Johnston C, Guttormsen AB and Nexo E (2006) Holotranscobalamin and total transcobalamin in human plasma: determination, determinants, and reference values in healthy adults. Clin Chem 52: 129–137

[121] Richardson DR and Ponka P (1997) The molecular mechanisms of the metabolism and transport of iron in normal and neoplastic cells. Biochim Biophys Acta 1331: 1–40

[122] Roberts AG, Whatley SD, Morgan RR, Worwood M and Elder GH (1997) Increased frequency of the haemochromatosis cys 282 tyr mutation in sporadic prophyria cutanea tarda. Lancet 349: 321–323

[123] Robinson SH (1990) Degradation of hemoglobin. In: Williams WJ, Beutler W, Erslev AJ and Lichtman MA (eds) Hematology, 4th edn. McGraw-Hill, New York

[124] Roth D, Smith RD, Schulman G, et al. (1994) Effects of recombinant human erythropoietin on renal function in chronic renal failure predialysis patients. Am J Kidney Dis 24: 777–784

[125] Sandborn WJ and Hanauer SB (1999) Antitumor necrosis factor therapy for inflammatory bowel disease: a review of agents, pharmacology, clinical results and safety. Inflamm Bowel Dis 5: 119–133

[126] Sassa S (1990) Synthesis of heme. In: Williams WJ, Beutler E, Erslev AJ and Lichtman MA (eds) Hematology, 4th edn. McGraw-Hill, New York, pp 332–335

[127] Schilling RE and Williams WJ (1995) Vitamin B12 deficiency: under-diagnosed, overtreated? Hosp Pract 30: 47–52

[128] Schulze-Osthoff K, Ferrari D, Los M, Wesselborg S and Peter ME (1998) Apoptosis signaling by death receptors. Eur J Biochem 254: 439–459

[129] Schurek HJ (1992) Oxygen shunt diffusion in renal cortex and its physiological link to erythropoietin production. In: Pagel H, Weiss C and Jelkmann W (eds) Pathophysiology and pharmacology of erythropoietin. Springer, Berlin Heidelberg New York Tokyo, pp 53–55

[130] Scigalla P, Ehmer B, Woll EM, et al. (1990) Zur individuellen Ansprechbarkeit terminal niereninsuffizienter Patienten auf die RhEPO-Therapie. Nieren-Hochdruckerkrankungen 19: 178–183

[131] Scott JM and Weir DG (1980) Drug induced megaloblastic change. Clin Haematol 9: 587–606

[132] Sears D (1992) Anemia of chronic disease. Med Clin North Am 76: 567–579

[133] Shapiro HM (1995) Practical flow cytometry, 3rd edn. Wiley-Liss, New York

[134] Shinozuka N, Koyama J, Anzai H, et al. (2000) Autologous blood transfusion in patients with hepatocellular carcinoma undergoing hepatectomy. Am J Surg 179: 42–45

[135] Sullivan JL (1996) Perspectives on the iron and heart disease debate. J Clin Epidermial 49: 1345–1352

[136] Sunder-Plassmann G and Hörl WH (1997) Erythropoietin and iron. Clin Nephrol 47: 141–157

[137] Suominen P, Punnonen P, Rajamaki A and Irjala K (1997) Evaluation of new immunoenzymometric assay for measuring soluble transferrin receptor to detect iron deficiency in anaemic patients. Clin Chem 43: 1641–1646

[138] Suominen P, Punnonen K, Rajamaki A and Irjala K (1998) Serum transferrin receptor and transferrin receptor-ferritin index identity healthy subjects with subclinical iron deficits. Blood 92: 2934–2939

[139] Thomas C and Thomas L (2007) Biochemical and hematoligical indices in the diagnosis of functional iron deficiency. Clin Chem 48: 1066–1076

[140] Thomas L (2005) Porphyrine. In: Thomas L (Hrsg) Labor und Diagnose, 6. Aufl. TH-Books, Frankfurt/Main, pp 646–659

[141] Thorpe SJ, Walker D, Arosio P, Heath A, Cook JD and Worwood M (1997) International collaborative study to evaluate a recombinant ferritin preparation as an international standard. Clin Chem 43: 1582–1587

[142] Thorstensen K and Romslo I (1993) The transferrin receptor: its diagnostic value and its potential as therapeutic target. Scand J Clin Lab Invest 53 (suppl 215): 113–120

[143] Tuomainen T, Punnonen K, Nyyssönen K and salvonen JT (1998) Association between body iron stores and the risk of myocardial infarction in men. Circulation 97: 1461–1466

[144] Valcour AA, Krzymowski G, Onoroski M, Bowers GN Jr and McComb RB (1990) Proposed reference method for iron in serum used to evaluate two automated iron methods. Clin Chem 36: 1789–1792

[145] Vanrenterghem Y, Barany P, Mann J and on behalf of the European/Australian NESP 970290 Study Group (2000) Novel erythropoiesis stimulating protein (NESP) maintains hemoglobin (Hgb) in ESRD patients when administered once weekly or once every other week. J Am Soc Nephrol 11 (suppl): A1365 (abstract)

[146] Volk HD, Keyßer G and Burmester GR (2007) Zytokine und Zy-tokinrezeptoren. In: Thomas L (ed) Labor und Diagnose, 6. Aufl. TH Books Verlagsgesellschaft, Frankfurt, pp 1039–1051

[147] Waheed A, Parkkila S, Saarnio J, et al. (1999) Association of HFE protein with transferrin receptor in crypt enterocytes of human duodenum. Proc Nat Acad Sci USA 96: 1579–1584

[148] Ware CF, Santee S and Glass E (1998) Tumor necrosis factor-relat-ed ligands and receptors. In: Thomson AW (ed) Cytokine hand-book. Academic Press, San Diego, pp 549–593

[149] Weiss G (1999) Iron and anemia of chronic disease. Kidney Int 55: 12–17

[150] Weiss G, Houston T, Kastner S, Johrer K, Grunewald K and Brock JH (1997) Regulation of cellular iron metabolism by erythropoi-etin: activation of iron-regulatory protein and upregulation of transferrin receptor expression in erythroid cells. Blood 89: 680–687

[151] Weiss G, Wachter H and Fuchs D (1995) Linkage of cell-mediated immunity to iron metabolism. Immunol Today 6: 495–500

[152] Weiss G, Werner-Felmayer G, Werner ER, Grunewald K, Wachter H and Hentze MW (1994) Iron regulates nitric oxide synthase ac-tivity by controlling nuclear transcription. J Exp Med 180: 969–976

[153] Witherspoon LR (1981) Vitamin B_{12}: Are serum radioassay mea-surements reliable? J Nuc Med 22: 474–477

[154] Yap GS and Stevenson MM (1994) Inhibition of in vitro erythro-poiesis by soluble mediators of Plasmodium chalandi AS malaria: lack of a major role of interleukin l, TNF-alpha and gamma-inter-feron. Infect Immun 62: 357–362

Further Reading

Andrews NC (1999) Disorders of iron metabolism. N Engl J Med 341: 1986–1995

Beck N (2009) Diagnostic hematology. Springer, Berlin

Crichton R (2009) Inorganic biochemistry of iron metabolism. From mo-lecular mechanisms to clinical consequences. Wiley, Chichester New York Weinheim Brisbane Singapore Toronto

Lichtman MA (2001) William's hematology, 6th edn. McGraw-Hill, New York

Malyszko J (2009) Hemojuvelin: the hepcidin story continues. Kidney Blood Press Res 32: 71–76

Meyers RA (ed) (2007) Immunology: from cell biology to disease. Wiley-VCH, Weinheim

Kidney Int 1999, Vol. 55, Suppl 69

Thomas L (ed) (2007) Labor und Diagnose, 7. Aufl. TH Books Verlagsgesellschaft, Frankfurt

Weiss G, Gordeuk VR, Heshko C (eds) (2005) Anemia of chronic diseases. CRC Press, Boca Raton, FL

Subject Index

Aceruloplasminemia 39, 144

Acute phase protein 26, 129, 143, 172

Acute phase reaction 27, 31, 47, 55, 64, 110

Agglutination 135

Alcoholism 6, 41, 114, 119, 121, 123, 153, 165

Anaphylactic reaction 78

Anemias 1, 2, 4, 5, 8, 14, 16, 18, 21, 22, 24–37, 40, 42–46, 48, 49, 52, 53, 55–61, 63, 64, 66–68, 70, 73, 74, 76–78, 80–110, 114, 116–120, 122–130, 150, 151, 163–171

  aplastic 35, 37, 90, 114, 116, 163

  chronic diseases (ACD) 29

  corpuscular 129

  hemolytic 35, 36, 44, 49, 117, 128, 129, 171

  hypochromic 25, 26, 28, 57, 60, 66, 70, 80–105, 165

  hyperchromic 42, 118, 119, 165

  iron deficient 32, 35, 60, 68, 70, 74, 77, 94

  in renal failure 24, 37, 64, 105, 107, 128, 150

  macrocytic 40, 42, 43, 53, 78, 117–119, 120, 122, 163, 165

  microcytic 26, 30, 44, 56, 58, 60, 66, 70, 117, 164, 165

  normocytic 32, 70, 91, 104, 106, 117, 126–128, 165

  pernicious 123–126, 164

  renal 21, 24, 30, 32, 33, 35, 37, 89, 90, 106–109, 117, 150

  sideroachrestic 45, 46

  spherocytic 48

  tumor anemias 28, 30, 52, 59, 80, 82, 90, 95, 98, 165

  WHO criteria 52

Anti-acute phase protein 28, 58

Antibody excess 136

Anulocytes 69, 70

Aplastic anemia 35, 37, 90, 114, 116, 163

Apoferritin 8, 9, 25

Apotransferrin 29, 86, 141

Ascorbic acid (Vitamin C) 4

Atherogenesis 79

Autoimmune diseases 49, 80, 101, 125

Automated cell count 153

Blood count 56, 61, 69, 75, 118, 122, 126, 132, 151–153, 157, 171

  large (red and white) 151

  small (red) 69, 75, 153

Blood donors 12, 26, 54, 59, 72, 79, 151

Bone marrow 1, 2, 8, 10–12, 15, 17–19, 22, 25, 30, 31, 35, 37, 40, 45, 48, 53, 54, 69, 82, 86, 87, 90, 93, 94, 97, 106, 107, 109, 117, 119, 120–122, 127, 155, 165–169

  stem cells 17, 109, 161

Borosilicate glass

  capillaries 160, 172

C1 units   41
Carboxyhemoglobin
    (COHb)   158
Cardiac muscle   137
Cardiovascular diseases   78
Cartilage   102
Ceruloplasmin (Endooxidase 1)
    4, 9, 39, 53, 85, 132, 144
CFU (colony forming unit)   19,
    20, 84, 162
Chronic renal insufficiency   22,
    89, 106–108, 150
Cobalamin (Vitamin B_{12})   17
Cold antibodies   128
Connective tissue   102
Continuous Erythropoiesis
    Receptor Activator
    (C.E.R.A.)   89
Cook's equation   109
Coombs test   49, 109
Coronary heart disease   79, 124
C-reactive protein (CRP)   31,
    27, 47, 55, 62–64, 81, 98,
    99, 102, 105, 108, 110,
    171–173
Cyanmethemoglobin   159
Cytokines   29, 60, 82–85, 87,
    90–93, 102–104, 172, 173
Cytotoxic effects   86

Darbopoietin alpha   88, 89, 100
5-Deoxyadenosylcobalamin   145
Deoxyhemoglobin   158
Diabetes mellitus   115, 125
Dialysis   32–34, 54, 55, 57, 60,
    61, 77–79, 89, 106–112, 116,
    120, 121, 129, 151, 170

Divalent metal transporter 1
    (DMT1, DCT1)   3, 4
Duodenum   4, 5, 74, 123

EDTA blood   156
Epoietin alpha, beta   88, 100
Erythroblasts   17, 45
Erythrocytes   9, 11–13, 17,
    20–22, 31–34, 42, 44–49, 52,
    64–66, 69, 90, 91, 93, 96,
    99– 109, 117, 122, 126, 127,
    129, 130, 142, 148, 152,
    155–157, 159–166, 168,
    170–172
    degradation   22
    hypochromic   31, 33, 99, 105,
        108, 164
    indices   66, 152
    maturation   64
    morphology   117
Erythrocyte sedimentation rate
    (ESR)   56, 81, 171, 172
Erythrocyte ferritin   170
Erythrocytopenia   162
Erythrocytosis   21, 22, 35, 36,
    150, 162
Erythropoiesis   13–15, 17–27,
    29–31, 33, 35–37, 40, 42, 45,
    48, 54, 55, 57–61, 63–66, 68,
    69, 76, 84–86, 88–91, 93, 94,
    101, 104, 106, 107, 108, 114,
    116–131, 161, 162, 165, 166,
    169, 170
    disturbances   40
Erythropoietin (EPO)   19, 35,
    66, 85, 132
    deficiency   21, 30, 33, 35, 60,
        96, 105, 117

determination   150
dose   94, 98, 110
recombinant human (rhu-
    EPO)   88, 89, 96, 98, 99,
    104, 105, 108, 110, 111, 150
Extrinsic factor   145

Ferric carboxymaltose   76
Ferritin   1, 4, 7–12, 14, 15, 22,
    24–29, 31–40, 46, 48, 50,
    52–65, 68–70, 72, 73, 75–77,
    79–81, 84, 86, 87, 91, 92, 95,
    97–99, 105, 107–113, 115, 119,
    132, 135, 137–140, 142–144,
    170
    apoferritin   8, 9, 25
    determination   34, 48, 54–56,
        59–61, 138
    isoferritin (acidic, basic)   8,
        10, 11, 22, 27, 59, 137, 138
    non-representative   31, 57,
        59, 119
    subunits   9, 10, 12, 137, 142,
        172
    synthesis   8, 25, 29, 58, 84
    clinical interpretation   91, 167
    ferritin release   29, 80
Ferrochelatase   46
Ferroportin   4, 5, 38, 114
Ferrous fumarate   75
Ferrous gluconate   75
Ferrous sulfate   75
Flow cytometry   153–156
Folic acid   17, 32, 40–43, 109,
    117, 120–123, 126, 132,
    147–149, 170
    antagonists   32, 41

deficiency   40–43, 109, 117,
    121–123, 148, 170
    requirement   121, 122
Functional iron deficiency   26,
    31–33, 59–61, 63, 64, 97–99,
    108, 109

Glucuronic acid   23
Glucose-6-phosphate-dehydroge-
    nase   48, 49, 128, 129

Haptoglobin   5, 9, 47, 48, 53, 85,
    106, 117, 127–129, 132,
    142–144
Heidelberger-Kendall curve   136
Hematocrit (Hct)   53, 75, 79, 90,
    91, 99, 105, 108, 132, 150–152,
    157, 159, 160, 162–164,
    167–169
Hematologic system diseases   93
Hematology analyzer   65, 151,
    160–163
Heme   4, 5, 8, 9, 18, 23, 32, 48,
    94, 143, 171
Hemiglobin   158, 159
Hemochromatosis   16, 24, 25,
    36–40, 50, 56, 57, 76, 114–116,
    144
    acquired   114
    primary   37, 38, 50, 57,
        114–116
    secondary   56, 57, 116
Hemoglobin (Hb)   3, 9, 11–13,
    17, 18, 22–24, 26, 31, 34, 36,
    42–44, 47–53, 56, 61, 63, 66,
    68, 69, 76, 79, 86, 90, 91, 93–95,
    98, 99, 105–109, 111, 112, 122,
    126–130, 132, 143, 150, 152,

157–159, 162–164, 166, 170, 171

degradation   22, 23

derivatives   158

determination   158, 159

electrophoresis   43, 44, 49, 130

free Hb   47, 48, 129, 143, 158

globin content   31, 42, 53, 63, 66, 152, 170

Hemoglobinopathies   43, 44, 48, 117, 130

Hemoglobinuria   48, 49, 128

Hemojuvelin   38, 114

Hemolysis   9, 22, 24, 25, 30, 35, 44, 46–49, 52, 53, 74, 93, 99, 106–108, 117, 121, 127–129, 134, 143, 165, 166, 169

autoimmune   30, 40, 49, 80, 101, 125, 128

corpuscular   44, 46, 48, 49, 129, 157, 162

extracorpuscular   46, 48, 128

Hemopexin   5, 9, 47, 48, 143

Hemosiderin   8, 9, 14, 50, 53, 54, 113

Hemosiderosis   37, 97

Hepcidin   3, 5, 16, 29, 30, 38, 100, 114

HFE gene   5, 38, 114

HFE protein   38, 114

HLA   38, 40, 114

Hodgkin's disease   97, 173

Homocysteine   42, 43, 120, 149, 150

Hyperhomocysteinemia   43

Hypermenorrhea   72

Hypoferremia   51

Impedance-based cell counters   156–158

Infections   27–29, 49, 54, 55, 57–59, 66, 78, 80, 88, 91, 95, 98, 101, 128, 173

Interferon (IFN)   29, 82–87, 94, 103

Interleukin-1 (IL-1)   84, 92, 101

Interleukin-6 (IL-6)   110, 171, 173

Interleukin-8 (IL-8)   171, 174

Intrinsic factor   17, 41, 123–126, 145, 146

Iron   1, 3–18, 22, 24–135, 137–144, 163–166, 170

absorption   3–5, 8, 22, 26, 33, 34, 38, 39, 45, 48, 50, 72, 75, 76, 114

administration   54, 68, 76, 77, 88

balance   5, 12, 24, 26, 39, 50, 68, 69, 105

binding proteins   135

circadian rhythm   133, 138, 140, 143

distribution   7, 8, 10, 27, 28, 32, 33, 40, 52, 53, 59–61, 66, 78, 80–105, 113, 141, 144, 165

deficiency   1, 4, 9, 12, 15, 24–33, 35, 39, 45, 50, 53–61, 63, 64, 68–80, 91, 92, 97–99, 108, 109, 113, 117, 126, 134, 141, 142, 163–165, 170

determination   8, 133

functional   26, 31–34, 57–61, 63, 64, 78, 97–100, 104, 108, 109

loss   12, 39, 48, 50, 75, 110,
    143
metabolism   1, 3–16, 24–67,
    84, 85, 99, 104, 110, 117,
    132, 140
overload   5, 7, 9, 14, 24, 25,
    27, 29, 30, 31, 33, 36–40, 44,
    45, 48, 53–57, 59, 61, 70, 85,
    108–111, 113–116, 141, 144
oxidation   39, 144
redistribution   1, 24, 25,
    28–31, 35, 53
requirement   4, 6–8, 12, 14,
    15, 22, 25, 27, 28, 33, 34, 50,
    51, 61, 71, 73, 76, 109,
saturation   7, 135
storage iron   1, 8, 9, 12, 25,
    50, 55, 56, 59, 60, 62, 63, 68,
    69, 85, 91, 137
storage tissues   137
therapy   27, 35, 36, 55–57, 75,
    76, 78, 79, 81, 86, 104, 105,
    108, 111
transport   4–6, 16, 28, 37, 69
transport iron   1, 12, 25, 26,
    28, 32–34, 51, 61, 109
uptake   4, 5, 13, 14, 29, 60,
    84, 86, 116
utilization   24, 26, 32, 33, 46,
    60, 82, 97, 105–112, 130
Iron absorption test   50
Iron-binding capacity   5–7, 132,
    135, 140, 141
    latent (LIBC)   7, 132, 135,
        140
    total (TIBC)   7, 132, 135, 140,
        141
Iron gluconate   75, 76

Iron saccharate   75–77, 110
Iron sulfate   75

Kidney   4, 21, 35, 52, 89, 90, 93,
    102, 106, 108, 150, 151, 165,
    171, 173

Lactic acid dehydrogenase
    (LDH)   47, 117, 128, 129
Low densitity lipoprotein
    (LDL)   36, 37
Lesch-Nyhan syndrome   126
Leukocyte dilution   158
Liver   4–12, 16, 17, 19, 22, 23,
    28, 35, 36, 38, 41, 46, 47, 53, 54,
    56, 57, 59, 69, 77, 80, 90,
    114–116, 124, 129, 137, 138,
    142, 143, 144, 145, 147, 151,
    165, 171, 172, 173
Lipopolysaccharide (LPS)   29,
    82, 86

Macrocytes   42
Macrophages   4, 16, 22, 29, 30,
    38, 46, 60, 82–84, 86–88, 91,
    92, 101–104, 174
Magnesium carbonate   135
Malaria   49, 129
Malignancy   28, 91, 92, 96, 121
Mean cellular hemoglobin
    content of erythrocytes (MCH)
    66, 69, 91, 106, 118, 126, 152,
    153, 157, 162–164, 165
Mean cellular hemoglobin
    concentration of erythrocytes
    (MCHC)   69, 152, 153, 157,
    162, 164, 165

Mean cell volume of erythrocytes (MCV) 24, 66, 69, 91, 106, 118, 152, 153, 157, 162–165

Mean platelet volume 153, 157

Megaloblastic anemias 57

Met-hemoglobin (Met Hb) 130

Methylmalonic acid 43, 132, 147

Microhematocrit method 160

Monocytes 36, 82, 85, 92, 101, 103, 104, 152, 153, 174

Mucosa cell 36

Myelodysplastic syndrome (MDS) 24, 31, 40, 57, 58, 64, 96, 97, 117

Myoglobin 12, 50–52

N-5-methyltetrahydrofolic acid (MTHFA) 147, 148

Neoplasias 27, 60, 93

NO (nitrogen oxide) 84, 86

Normoblasts 17
  basophilic 17
  oxyphilic 17

Novel erythropoiesis stimulating protein (NESP) 88

Orotic acid 119, 126

Oxygen radicals 36

Oxyhemoglobin 158

Pannus 102

Parietal cells 17, 125

Particle count 157, 158

Pentraxin 172

Phagocytosis 22, 36, 162

Phlebotomy 55, 115

Porphyrin 23, 32, 34, 45, 46, 145, 171

Placenta 10, 11, 16

Polycythemia 21, 35, 90, 130

Proerythroblasts 17, 20

Pteromylonoglutaminic acid (PGA) 147

Red blood cell count (RBC) 75, 148, 152, 153, 156, 157, 161, 162, 166, 168

Red blood cell indices 162–165

Reticulocyte 14, 17, 18, 24, 30, 31, 33, 48, 53, 63, 65, 66, 91, 97, 99, 105–107, 109, 118, 122, 126, 127, 142, 152, 155, 156, 165–170
  Hb content 170
  production index (RPI) 53, 105, 168, 169

Reticulocyte count 14, 18, 30, 33, 53, 65, 66, 106, 107, 126, 127, 142, 152, 165–170

Reticuloendothelial system (RES) 21, 22, 54, 56, 85, 87, 90, 91, 104, 110, 115, 116, 129, 162

Rheumatoid arthritis (RA) 78, 80, 88, 91, 101–104

Serum amyloid A (SAA) 110, 171

Sickle cell anemia 43, 48, 49, 130

Soluble transferrin receptor (sTfR) 3, 7, 14, 15, 25, 26, 30, 34, 35, 52–54, 59, 68, 69, 91, 92, 98, 99, 107, 109, 132, 138, 142

Stem cells 17, 109, 161

Target cells   44, 49, 130, 150
Tetrahydrofolic acid (THFA)
   41, 120, 123, 147, 148
Thalassemia   36, 43, 44, 45, 48,
   58, 64, 114, 116, 117, 130, 164,
   165
Thrombosis   173
Thrombocyte count   97
Tissue hypoxia   20, 30
Transcobalamin   123, 132, 145,
   146, 147
Transferrin   3–7, 12–15, 17, 22,
   24–31, 33–40, 51–54, 56–61,
   68, 69, 79, 81, 84–88, 91, 92,
   97–99, 104, 107, 109, 111, 114,
   115, 132, 133, 135, 136,
   138–144, 170
Transferrin receptor   3, 5, 7,
   12–15, 17, 24–26, 28–30,
   33–38, 52–54, 59–61, 68, 69,
   84, 86–88, 91, 92, 97–99, 104,
   107, 109, 114, 132, 138, 142
Transferrin saturation   5, 7,
   13, 24–29, 31, 33, 34, 37–40,
   52, 53, 56–59, 61, 68, 69, 79, 81,
   91, 92, 98, 99, 109, 111, 115,
   132, 135, 141, 144, 170

Tumor anemias   28, 30, 52, 59,
   80, 82, 90, 95, 98, 165
Tumor necrosis factor-α
   (TNF-α)   29, 83, 84, 86, 87,
   92, 94, 101, 103, 171, 175
Tumor Necrosis factor receptor
   Fc fusion proteins   92

Uroporphyria   46

Vitamin B$_{12}$ 17, 32, 40–43, 46,
   52, 53, 72, 99, 105, 109, 117,
   119–126, 132, 145–149, 165,
   166, 170

Warm antibodies   128

Zinc protoporphyrin   34, 171
Zollinger-Ellison syndrome   126